allergy-free
LIVING

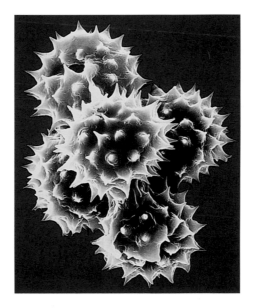

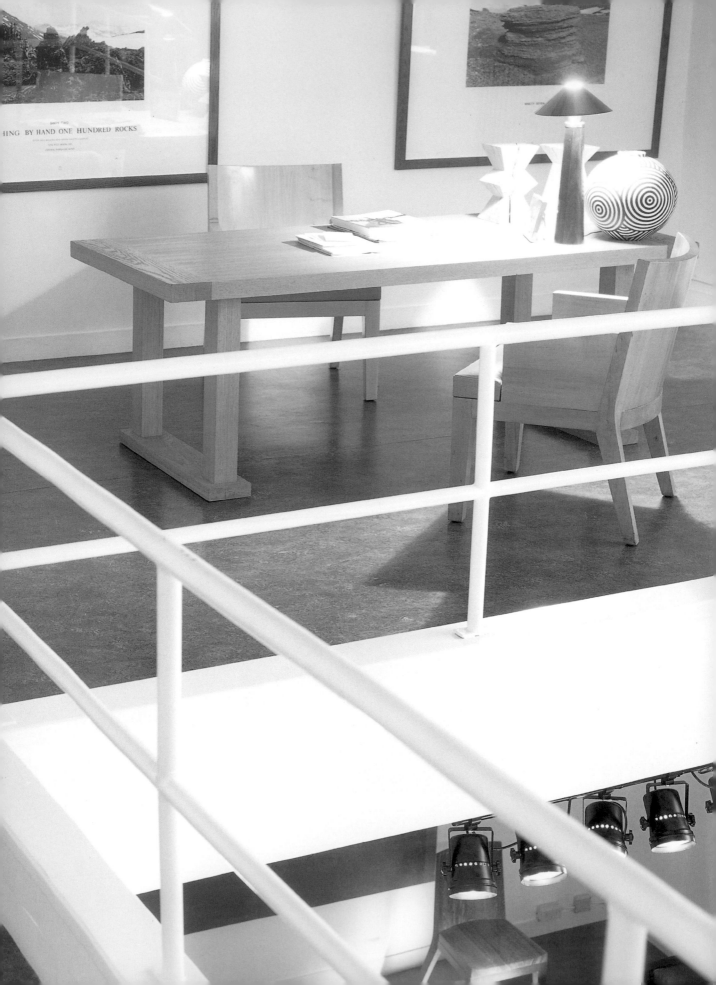

allergy-free LIVING

How to create a healthy, allergy-free home and lifestyle

DR PETER HOWARTH AND ANITA REID

MITCHELL BEAZLEY

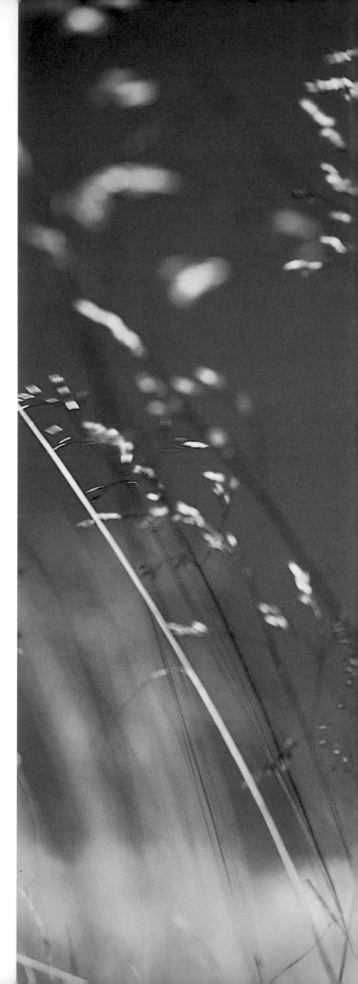

To my husband Nevile, and my parents, Annie and Lawrence,
Anita Reid

To Susan, Sally, and Joanna, **Peter Howarth**

First published in Great Britain in 2000
by Mitchell Beazley,
an imprint of Octopus Publishing Group Limited
2–4 Heron Quays, London E14 4JP
Reprinted 2000
Executive Editor **Judith More**
Executive Art Editor **Janis Utton**
Project Editors **Julia North, Selina Mumford**
Editor **Jonathan Hilton**
Designed by **Lovelock & Co.**
Picture Researcher **Helen Stallion**
Production Controllers **Rachel Staveley, Nancy Roberts**

A CIP record for this book is available from
the British Library.

ISBN 1 84000 233 6

The publishers have made every effort to ensure
that all instructions given in this book are accurate and
safe, but they cannot accept liability for any resulting
injury, damage, or loss to either person or property
whether direct or consequential and howsoever arising.
The author and publishers will be grateful for any
information which will assist them in keeping future
editions up to date.

Printed in China by Toppan Printing Co Ltd

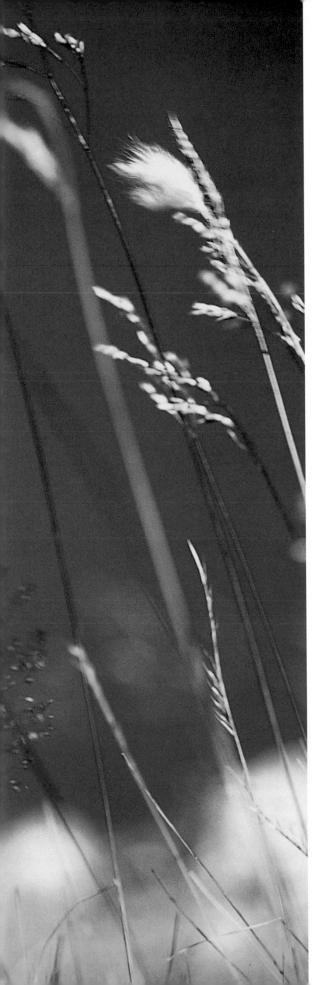

Contents

6   Introduction

10 **UNDERSTANDING YOUR ALLERGY**

12 What is an Allergy?

24 Contributory Factors

44 Diagnosis and Management

48 **THE ALLERGY-FREE HOME**

50 Indoor Air Quality

60 Heating

62 Floors and Walls

66 Home Improvements

70 Furnishings and Fixtures

72 Cleaning Your Home

78 THE IDEAL ROOM

80 The Ideal Bedroom

86 The Ideal Children's Room

90 The Ideal Living Room

94 The Ideal Kitchen

100 The Ideal Bathroom

104 The Ideal Home Office

106 The Ideal Conversion

110 Outside the Home

114 CASE HISTORIES

116 Building from Scratch

118 Case History 1

124 Case History 2

130 Directory of Suppliers and Organisations

135 Glossary

138 Bibliography

139 Index

143 Acknowledgments

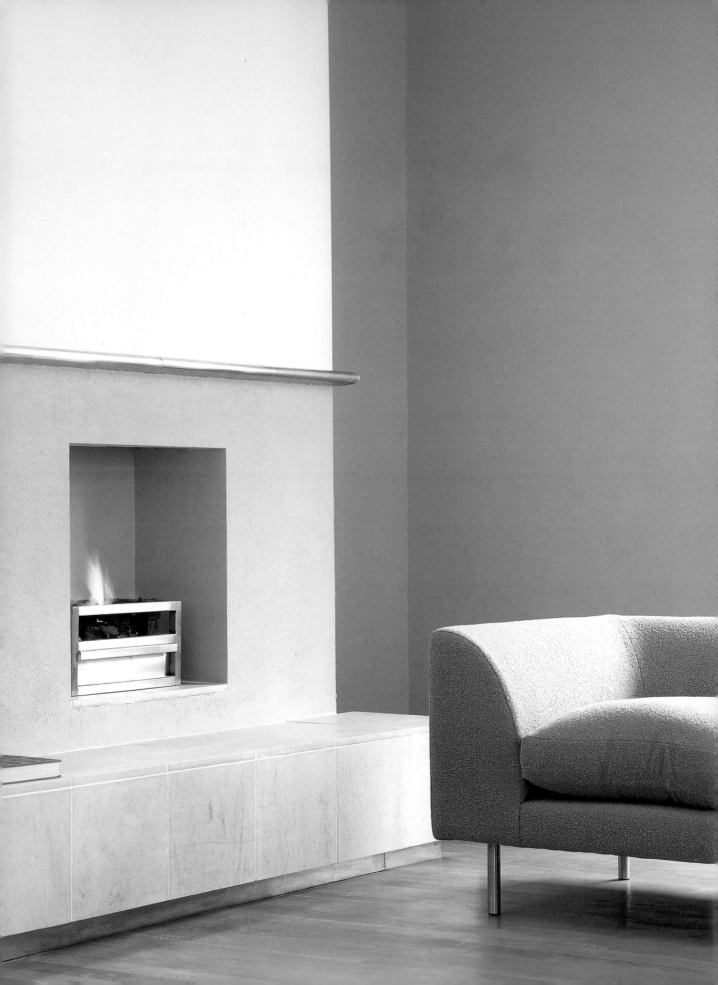

Introduction

We are all becoming increasingly aware of allergies and the problems that they represent in the daily lives of many people. This is due partly to the publicity given to the tragic, fatal cases involving severe reactions, such as peanut allergy leading to anaphylaxis, and partly to the increased media coverage of the much more common diseases associated with allergy, such as asthma, hay fever, and eczema. This heightened public interest and awareness is in the context of a significant increase over the last 40 or 50 years in the number of individuals who suffer from allergic problems. This increase is most striking in the more affluent countries of the world, and in these countries allergic diseases are the commonest chronic conditions that impair quality of life and require medical treatment. For example, a recent international survey has revealed that approximately one in three 13 to 14 year-olds living in the United Kingdom have symptoms consistent with asthma, while one in four of the same adolescent population in the United States is similarly affected. Thus, combatting allergy has become one of the major health challenges facing the developed world.

The underlying basis for the rise in the numbers of allergy sufferers has been the focus of considerable research. Much of this attention has concentrated on the quality of the outdoor air we breathe, especially as the roads have become more and more congested with traffic generating a cocktail of exhaust pollutants. Although there still remains some uncertainty over a possible contribution from diesel exhaust particulates, research has identified that sources of air pollution outside the home cannot account for the increasing prevalence of allergy, and so other reasons have to be investigated. Careful evaluation of individuals with asthma, eczema, and rhinitis has discovered a significant allergic tendency within these groups of people. This tendency is predominantly linked to the allergens commonly found within the home environment, such as those related to house-dust mites, cockroaches, domestic pets, and, to a lesser extent, moulds. Exposure to these allergens induces inflammation, and can explain the cause and the persistence of these diseases. Therefore, researchers' attention is now much more focused on the interior environment and those factors that influence the presence and level of interior allergens, as well as the presence of pollutants in buildings that, through their irritant effects, worsen the symptoms of allergies. This focus is clearly relevant once you realize that many people now spend from 75 to 90 percent of their time inside, most within their own homes.

About this book

So you or someone in your family suffers from an allergy and you want to know more about it? Turn to the first section of this book, which defines commonly used terms and explains what allergy is and how it leads to the range of problems people experience. Common allergic conditions such as asthma, hay fever, rhinitis, eczema, and urticaria, as well as anaphylaxis, are all clearly explained and looked at in relationship to exposure to the airborne, ingested, or contact allergens underlying these conditions. These allergens are discussed in detail, providing insight into the environments and conditions that favour them. Details are also given of the common allergens found outside, such as the tree, grass, or weed pollens that largely contribute to seasonal rhinitis, conjunctivitis, and asthma. In addition, there is a discussion of the sources and effects of interior pollutants in allergic individuals, and how the effects of these pollutants contrast with exterior ones. This section also discusses approaches to the diagnosis and treatment of allergic diseases. This will help you to understand why your doctor has chosen a particular approach to your treatment, such as allergen avoidance, desensitizing injections, or drug treatment. By the nature of the book, this aspect is not comprehensive, but it does put allergen avoidance, about which much of the book is concerned, into perspective.

So how do I avoid allergens? The first section of this book provides the background for the subsequent sections, which reveal a wealth of practical information about the home environment and the steps that you can take to improve it for people with allergies.

The second section looks at the home in relationship to heating, lighting, cooking, ventilation, furnishing, floor covering, and cleaning. Each part explores in detail the range of approaches or products available and considers the advantages and disadvantages of their use, either in relationship to their influence on interior allergens or their potential as a source of irritant chemicals or gases. This information is integrated so that you can make informed decisions when it comes to selecting household appliances and furnishings.

The third part of the book, *The Ideal Room*, visits each room within the average home and details the specific changes that can be made to lessen your exposure to allergens within that room. The easy-to-use bullet point guide for each room not only highlights problem areas, it also prioritizes the changes that can be undertaken. Any alterations have to be balanced against the impact they might have on the comfort factor within your home, and not all adaptations may be acceptable, or indeed necessary, for every individual. This part of the book has been extended to include very useful coverage concerning the ideal conversion, since these days it is increasingly common for people to convert their attics or basements to make new living areas, rather than move house, when extra space becomes necessary.

Thus, by referring to the index or by using the cross-references within the text, you should readily be able to find information relating to any specific room you wish to modify or find details concerning specific aspects of your living environment.

The final section of the book describes initiatives that have been undertaken around the world to provide low-allergen housing for people with allergic diseases, including that by the American Lung Association. It also details actual case histories of people who have built low-allergen houses and the impact that these have had on their lives and their allergies.

Among the first low-allergen house initiatives was The Healthy Building Project in Denmark, as was The National Asthma Campaign Low Allergen House in the United Kingdom, which was open to the public for the Future World Exhibition in 1994. This initiative followed on from the National Asthma Campaign Low Allergen Garden, which was instigated by Selina Thistleton-Smith along with her sister, the garden designer Lucy Huntington, and was the basis for the book *Creating a Low-Allergen Garden*. Selina, along with the late John Donaldson, who sadly died from his asthma, were the major driving forces in encouraging the National Asthma Campaign initiative. This involved several people, with one of the authors of this book, Dr Peter Howarth, acting as medical advisor to the project.

The home received substantial publicity at the time of the exhibition, and many of the considerations that went into planning the design of that house have been incorporated into the content of this book. What became immediately apparent from talking to visitors to the house was the desire on the part of many people to undertake the management of their disease and to do something to help themselves, rather than having to depend on medication. Another fact that emerged from the visitors to the low-allergen house was the deficiency in practical advice available to those wishing to avoid allergens in the home.

By collecting all this information together in this book, we hope to be able to provide for the first time a comprehensive and easy-to-use guide to what practically can be done by individuals with allergic diseases to modify their home environment and to help reduce the burden and severity of their condition.

The diagram below illustrates some of the more common sources of allergens and irritants within and around the home.

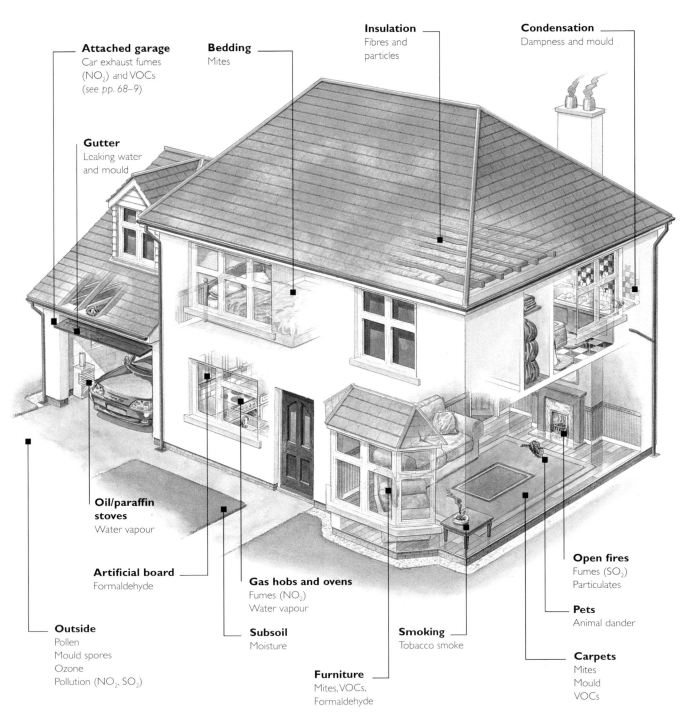

Attached garage
Car exhaust fumes
(NO_2) and VOCs
(*see pp. 68–9*)

Bedding
Mites

Insulation
Fibres and
particles

Condensation
Dampness and mould

Gutter
Leaking water
and mould

Oil/paraffin stoves
Water vapour

Artificial board
Formaldehyde

Outside
Pollen
Mould spores
Ozone
Pollution (NO_2, SO_2)

Gas hobs and ovens
Fumes (NO_2)
Water vapour

Subsoil
Moisture

Furniture
Mites, VOCs,
Formaldehyde

Smoking
Tobacco smoke

Open fires
Fumes (SO_2)
Particulates

Pets
Animal dander

Carpets
Mites
Mould
VOCs

Understanding Your Allergy

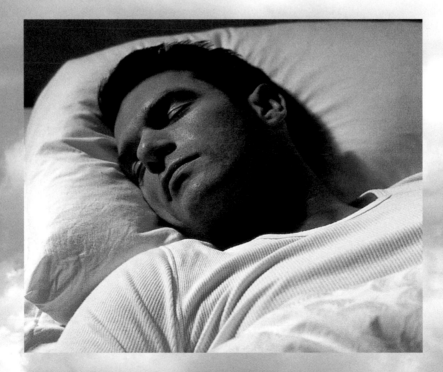

What is an Allergy?

Each of you reading this book will have your own idea of what an allergy is. In very simple terms, an allergy is an adverse reaction. You will often hear people say things such as "I'm allergic to cats", or "I'm allergic to this or that type of food", or even "I'm allergic to Monday mornings". In all these instances, the implication is that contact with whatever they are expressing concern about causes them some sort of unpleasant or adverse feeling or reaction.

When the term "allergy" was first coined in the early years of the twentieth century by the Austrian physician Clemens Freiherr von Pirquet, the word was used to mean a change – either good or bad – in the way that the body reacted. A good reaction provided immunity, while a bad one produced hypersensitivity (see opposite). Over the years, the term "allergy" has come to be associated solely with immune hypersensitivity reactions, whereas the term "immunity" is linked to the body's beneficial immune responses.

Why do allergic reactions occur?

An adverse immune response is the body's attempt to kill or expel a foreign protein that has invaded it. From the body's perspective, therefore, an allergic reaction is a protective mechanism. While immune reactions can occur in response to viruses or bacteria – and, on occasions, inappropriately to the body's own proteins – allergic reactions usually occur in response to external, non-infectious substances.

When these protective reactions are directed against what are basically harmless proteins, it is the allergic reaction itself – rather than the external agent it is directed against – that becomes the focus of the problem. Most of the allergies that trouble people today fall into this category.

Which parts of the body are affected?

Allergic reactions tend to occur in the parts of the body where the immune system is activated. Thus, airborne proteins that are inhaled cause reactions in the nose and airways of the lung (see diagrams below). If these airborne proteins also settle on the surface of the eye, then symptoms may also arise there. Proteins that are eaten will either cause a gastrointestinal upset or, if they are absorbed into the blood, they have the potential to cause a variety of symptoms involving the skin, joints, cardiovascular, and central nervous systems, as well as the nose and lungs.

Similar responses can occur with foreign proteins that are injected into the body, such as stings from bees or wasps, for example. Although the skin is an obvious site for contact, the barrier function of the skin protects the immune system from exposure unless it is damaged by the protein or the protein contains enzymes that

THE AIRWAYS UNDER ATTACK

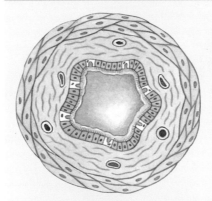

In a normal airway, as represented by this cross-section, air passes easily up and down the bronchial tubes as you breathe. The outer layer of muscle is relaxed and there is no swelling of the inner lining of the tube itself.

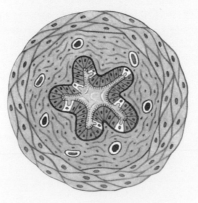

The asthmatic airway looks very different. Most obviously, the tube has become narrowed, and this makes breathing more difficult. The muscle around the outside is thicker and the lining of the airway is swollen due to inflammation. Increased amounts of mucus are being secreted into the airway, which contribute to the blocking of the breathing tubes. These changes are brought on by allergy.

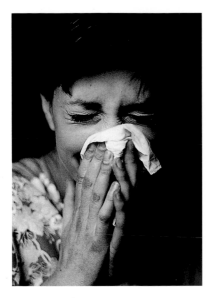

An allergy that causes rhinitis (or nasal inflammation) will result in bouts of frequent sneezing as well as a runny or blocked nose.

or possibly following its absorption from the mucous membranes of the eye, nose, or lungs.

The immune system reacts to the presence of a foreign protein by producing an area of inflammation (*see below*). This happens when special immune cells within the affected tissue become activated. These immune cells release chemicals, and it is these that give rise to the localized symptoms you experience. This inflammation is often signified by the suffix "itis" that is added to the name of the organ involved, such as "dermatitis", "sinusitis", or "conjunctivitis".

What is inflammation?

Your body's immune responses are designed to protect you by killing or expelling the carrier of any foreign protein that is perceived as "attacking" the body. With an infection, this protective response kills the bacteria and so the response terminates itself. The local response involved in this

process causes swelling, redness, pain, and an increase in the blood flow – this is why the swollen part of your body feels hot. This process, which involves the recruitment of white blood cells (known as neutrophil white cells) from the circulatory system, is called "inflammation".

With an allergic reaction, a similar, but lesser, inflammation occurs. However, since the proteins, or allergens, to which you are sensitized are inert (rather than alive, as bacteria are) and are associated with the environment you are in, this type of inflammation is persistent and results in the symptoms you experience.

In contrast to your body's immune responses to fight bacteria, in which the neutrophil white cell is recruited to combat the infection, in an allergic response another type of white cell, an eosinophil white cell, is recruited. A different type of white cell is involved because the immune response to allergens is different to that against infection.

enable it to penetrate the skin. Although it is easy to assume that an allergic reaction involving the skin is some sort of contact allergy, it could, in fact, be a response to a foreign protein that has entered the blood's circulation system after being ingested,

COMMONLY USED TERMS

Any discussion of allergies involves terms with which you may not be familiar. Those defined below may help (*see also Glossary, pp. 136–8*).

Allergy A condition in which an *allergen* induces an immune response in the body that is associated with the increased production of an antibody, known as *immunoglobulin E*, which leads to symptoms and specific diseases, such as asthma or hay fever.

Allergen An intrinsically harmless substance that induces an allergic-type immune response in predisposed individuals.

Immunoglobulin E (IgE) An antibody that is associated with an allergic immune response. This

antibody is usually present in the body only in tiny amounts. However, people with a genetic predisposition to increased IgE production overproduce this antibody on exposure to allergens. Such people are termed *atopic*.

Atopy A positive response to tests for increased *IgE* production is indicative of atopy. Atopy tends to run in families, but is not always associated with symptoms of allergic disease. *Allergen* avoidance may convert an atopic person from an *allergy* sufferer to a symptom-free one.

Allergic hypersensitivity The adverse response of the immune system when it generates excess *IgE* in response to an allergen and gives rise to allergic reactions. The response to allergen exposure is retained within the immune

memory and, with repeated exposure, the reaction to that allergen can become more severe. This incremental response will be prevented by allergen avoidance. Allergic hypersensitivity is an adverse form of immunity.

Immunity Describes the activation of the immune system to generate protective antibodies against foreign proteins (usually infections) and the retention of this response information in the immune memory, so that if that protein is encountered again, the body responds rapidly. This immunity can be acquired naturally through infection or can be induced through vaccination. The antibodies generated in the protective response (immunoglobulins) are of a different type to those involved in allergy.

AIRBORNE ALLERGIES

Allergy-inducing particles of protein in the air commonly affect the nose, lower airways (lungs), and eyes. One of our first lines of defence against these agents is, in fact, the nose, which is an important filter, preventing many of the particles you breathe in from reaching your lungs. The filtering effect of the nose is due to a co-ordinated beating of invisibly small hairs, called cilia, which trap individual particles in the airstream as it passes over them. Not all particles are removed, however, and enough reach the lower airways to cause problems in many people. Reactions in different sites of the body are often linked. For example, asthma,

an allergic reaction in the lungs, and allergic nasal problems (rhinitis) commonly co-exist, as do rhinitis and allergic eye disease (conjunctivitis). Roughly 70 percent of patients with asthma also have rhinitis, and 30–40 percent of rhinitis sufferers also have asthma.

Asthma

This condition, which arises due to inflammation of the airways, is a very common one, and the number of people suffering from it is on the increase. A recent survey identified that about 35 percent of all 13–14 year olds in the United Kingdom have symptoms compatible with asthma,

while in the USA the figure is about 22.5 percent. Symptoms commonly associated with asthma include:
● Breathlessness
● A tight feeling in the chest
● Wheezy breathing
● Coughing

These symptoms, which are related to a narrowing of the airways, are not constant, however, and they are also variable in nature.

The onset of asthma commonly takes place in childhood, but it can start at any age. For most children with asthma (about 80 percent), and for more than half the adult sufferers,

Air passage from the nose

Breathing through the nose protects the lower airways, since particles in the air, such as allergens, are deposited on the lining of the nose. The inhaled air has to go through 180° in order to enter the windpipe. With mouth breathing, as occurs when the nose is blocked by allergic problems such as hay fever, this protective function is lost.

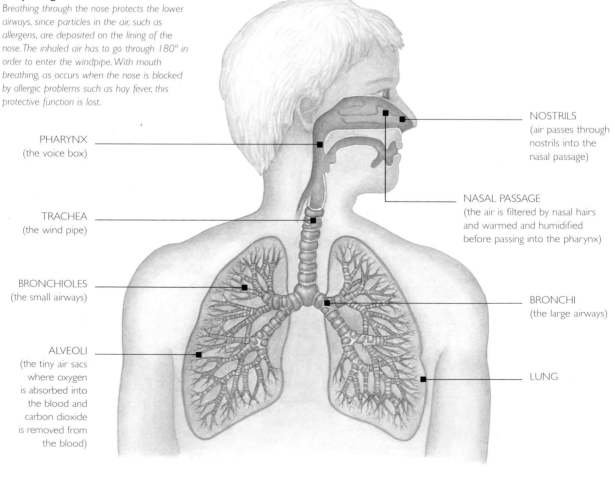

PHARYNX
(the voice box)

TRACHEA
(the wind pipe)

BRONCHIOLES
(the small airways)

ALVEOLI
(the tiny air sacs where oxygen is absorbed into the blood and carbon dioxide is removed from the blood)

NOSTRILS
(air passes through nostrils into the nasal passage)

NASAL PASSAGE
(the air is filtered by nasal hairs and warmed and humidified before passing into the pharynx)

BRONCHI
(the large airways)

LUNG

there is an allergic basis for their disease – this means that being in contact with a specific allergen makes their symptoms worse. This exposure may occur only periodically, such as when you visit the home of a cat-owning friend, or it can be continuous, as with the allergens resident in your home. Common allergens in the home are those relating to house-dust mites (see pp. 36–7), cockroaches (see pp. 38–9), and to pets (see pp. 40–1).

Continuous exposure to allergens in the home produces inflammation within the airways and makes them hyper-responsive to certain stimuli in the environment. These stimuli are called "trigger factors", since they temporarily trigger symptoms in those who already have asthma but do not actually induce the disease in the first place or maintain it, as allergens do. Common trigger factors include cold air, exercise, strong smells (such as perfume), cigarette smoke, aerosol sprays (such as hair sprays or furniture polish), and irritant gases (such as car exhaust fumes). Reactions to these types of factors do not represent an allergy, since they are irritants and your body's reaction does not involve the immune system. If you can manage to avoid allergens you will reduce the inflammation and by doing so lessen your response to any trigger factors you encounter.

Hay fever

This term describes the seasonal allergic response to pollen (see pp. 28–31) – usually grass, but also some

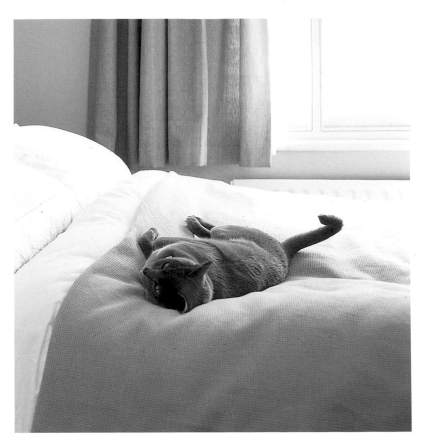

Pet allergy, particularly to allergens derived from the domestic cat, is an important cause of such conditions as asthma, rhinitis, and conjunctivitis.

weed and tree pollens. As hay fever is not due to hay, and is not generally associated with fever, it is a misnomer. The term has been kept, however, as it is readily understood.

Allergic responses to pollens occur most commonly in the nose (rhinitis) and eyes (conjunctivitis), and less commonly within the lower airways (asthma). The tendency to develop asthma depends on the level of the pollen count and the size of the pollen. Smaller pollens, such as birch (*Betula*) pollen, cause more asthma since more pollen grains are inhaled into the lower airways than with larger pollens, such as those from grasses. The associated inflammation of the nose and eyes commonly produces such symptoms as:

- Nasal itching
- Frequent sneezing
- Runny or blocked nose
- Itchy, watery, red eyes

Since pollen is seasonal, symptoms are present only for specific parts of the year. People with hay fever may also experience an itchy throat and roof of the mouth, an itchy sensation inside the ears, and sometimes a skin rash on contact with plants (such as grass).

Hay fever is on the increase, with about 25–30 percent of the adolescent population experiencing hay-fever symptoms. The timing of these symptoms will vary depending on the season of the year when the pollens are present. But since hay fever can have serious effects on sleep patterns, the ability to concentrate, and on work efficiency, it may have a negative impact on examination results and on performance during a range of outdoor sporting activities.

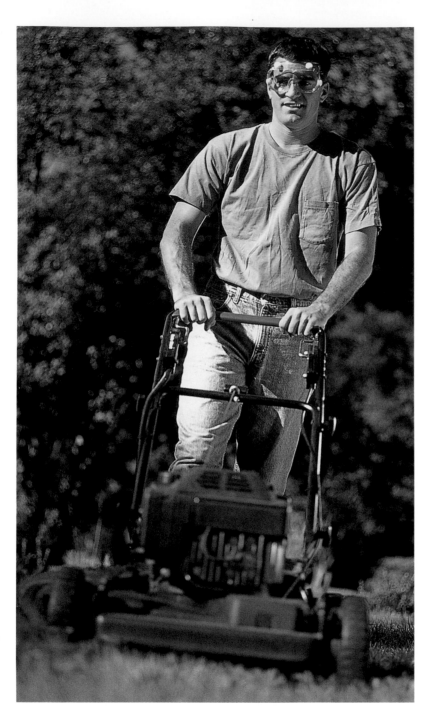

Wearing eye protection when cutting the grass can help to prevent the development of troublesome and irritating eye symptoms in hay-fever sufferers.

be associated with other symptoms, such as headaches, a loss of smell, and impaired taste. Perennial rhinitis is often associated with asthma. A blocked nose may lead to constant mouth-breathing, which can disturb sleep and worsen asthma. Poor sleep may impair daytime performance.

Conjunctivitis

Allergic conjunctivitis occurs when airborne allergens to which you are sensitized settle on the lining of your eye and start an immune reaction at that specific site. You will notice an inflammation of the inside of the eyelids, caused by the local release of chemicals. These chemicals act on the nerves and blood vessels to give rise to such commonly experienced symptoms as:

- Itchy eyes
- Watery eyes
- Reddening of the eyes
- Swelling of the eyelids

The most common allergy associated with the eye is seasonal allergic conjunctivitis, which is caused by an allergic reaction to tree, grass, or weed pollen. This occurs mainly in children and young adults and it is usually associated with rhinitis. The time of year for seasonal allergic conjunctivitis depends on the type of sensitization and when pollination occurs (see pp. 28–9).

Perennial allergic conjunctivitis is similar to the seasonal disease, except that it occurs all year around. This disease tends to be less severe than its seasonal counterpart and it is most commonly experienced in the early-to-

Rhinitis

People with allergic rhinitis may experience symptoms all year around (perennial) or only at certain times of the year (seasonal). Rhinitis is characterized by such symptoms as:

- Itchy nose
- Repeated sneezing
- Running or dripping nose
- Nasal congestion

Perennial rhinitis is usually linked with exposure to household allergens, such as that from house-dust mites, animals (see pp. 40–1), and cockroaches (see pp. 38–9). The daily symptoms are often identified as a "permanent cold".

With severe allergic rhinitis, the swelling of the lining of the nose, which occurs due to the inflammation produced by the allergic reaction, may

late teenage years. Almost 80 percent of sufferers are allergic to house-dust allergens and around 33 percent will suffer from rhinitis. Household allergens are, therefore, the major cause of perennial allergic conjunctivitis.

Neither seasonal nor perennial conjunctivitis poses any threat to eyesight and so treatment is usually based on relieving the symptoms reported by sufferers. There is, however, one form of allergic conjunctivitis that can threaten your eyesight – *vernal keratoconjunctivitis*. This is an extremely rare condition, and it accounts for a mere 0.1–0.5 percent of all eye disease. It mainly affects males (85 percent of cases) between the ages of 3 and 25 years living in hot, dry countries. Additional symptoms of this disease include:

● Photophobia – a painful reaction of the eye to light
● Spasms of the eyelids
● Blurring of vision
● Stringy discharge from the eyes

Allergic alveolitis

Small particles of protein in the air, around one-tenth the size of a small pinhead, travel down the airways and right out to the edge of the lungs to the alveoli, where oxygen from inhaled air is absorbed into the blood stream (*see p. 14*). An allergic reaction at this site, known as allergic alveolitis, interferes with the ability of the body to absorb oxygen, and so the oxygen level in the blood falls. With less oxygen available for the muscles, sufferers feel breathless and tired and have a cough. The allergic reaction to such small particles is different from

other forms of allergy, and with this type of immune response the person affected will experience the following symptoms:
● Feeling generally unwell
● Fever
● Headache
● Muscle aches and pains

Characteristically, the symptoms are noticed only hours after exposure and they may last for several days. With repeated exposure, however, the

disease becomes chronic and leads to permanent lung damage.

Allergens that produce allergic alveolitis have been linked with birds (budgerigars and pigeons) and with a variety of spores present in mouldy hay, straw, and compost. This condition is extremely rare compared with other allergic diseases caused by inhaling protein particles and spores, but it is important to be aware of it because of the potential lung damage it can cause.

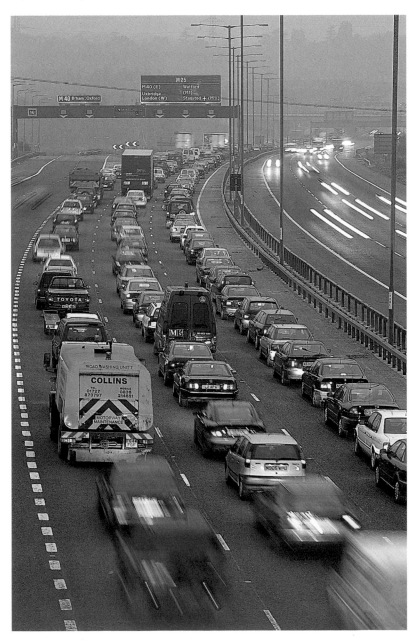

The cocktail of chemicals and particulates contained in road-traffic pollution (see pp. 32–3) is a factor that may worsen symptoms for hay-fever sufferers.

CONTACT ALLERGIES

If your skin reacts adversely to direct contact with something in the environment, it could be an allergic response (one involving the immune system) or a non-allergic response (due to an irritant). These conditions often co-exist, however, for example, damage to the skin by an allergen increases the likelihood of you responding to an irritant. The common skin conditions associated with contact responses are eczema and urticaria. Eczema is also called dermatitis (inflammation in the skin), and when an allergen is involved it is termed allergic contact dermatitis. (In the USA eczema is classified as atopic dermatitis, see p. 21.)

Allergic contact dermatitis

The development of this disease is brought about by repeated exposure to an allergen, which then leads to sensitization. Since the skin is an effective barrier to proteins entering the body, most cases of allergic contact dermatitis are caused by chemicals or metals entering the skin and binding to the body's own proteins and inducing an immune response. Symptoms are delayed and usually peak somewhere between 24 and 48 hours after exposure – so this is not an acute allergic reaction. Coming into contact with a large range of chemicals and metals can result in allergic contact dermatitis, although most are usually encountered only in a work environment. Contact with allergens in the home commonly affects the hands, face, and neck. Skin symptoms to look out for include:

● Reddening
● Swelling
● Intense itching
● Small bumps that may blister and weep
● Cracking, scaling, and thickening of the skin after repeated exposure

The list of potential causes of allergic contact dermatitis is extensive, but the metals, fragrances, and chemicals found in the following products and plants are common offenders:

● Cosmetics and face creams
● Perfumes
● Shampoos
● Nail varnish
● Hair dyes, perms, and setting agents
● Jewellery containing nickel
● Watch straps or buttons
● Poison ivy and poison oak

You may become aware of nickel sensitivity on your earlobes if you constantly wear earrings containing this metal. Unpleasant reactions can also occur in response to the chemicals found in some types of clothing dye. Those found in socks and shoe leather will affect your feet or the lower part of your legs.

Symptoms of irritant dermatitis are commonly experienced on your hands from contact with:

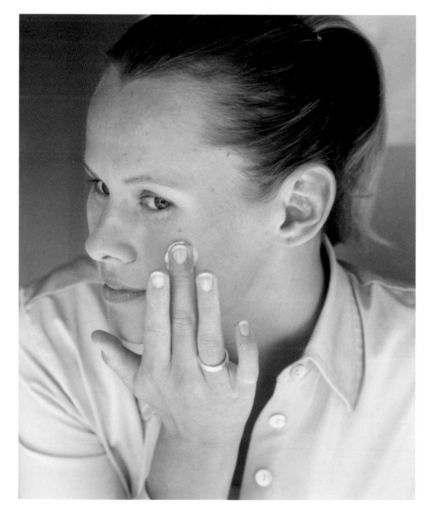

The chemicals contained in many brands of proprietary face creams and other cosmetic products may be important causes of skin rashes and irritation.

- Soaps
- Biological detergents
- Solvents
- Oil
- Alkalis, such as bleach

Although the reactions to allergic and irritant dermatitis may be difficult to differentiate, the principle of management remains the same: first, recognize the problem and determine what is causing it; and, second, avoid the offending agent in future.

Among plant sources of chemicals that could produce allergic contact dermatitis are the primulas. The chemical primin found in these plants (*see right*), especially *Primula obconica* and, to a lesser extent, *P. malacoides*, has a strong sensitizing potential and produces symptoms on the hands or arms or, indeed, anywhere you spread the contamination by touch.

Three other plants, poison ivy, poison oak, and poison sumak contain the chemical urushiol in their resin, which is a potent sensitizer. These plants are are all members of the genus *Toxicodendron*. Anybody who is sensitive to poison ivy, oak, or sumak may also react to other plants in the same family (Anacardiaccae), including cashews, mango, ginko, and Japanese lacquer.

Contact urticaria

With contact urticaria, you first experience reddened, itching skin, followed by a raised swollen area (hive), which is red initially but may then become pale in colour.

This condition is sometimes called hives, or nettle rash, since the reaction does resemble a nettle sting. Symptoms vary from very mild (with just a burning, mild itch) to severe (with extensive, itchy hives over all

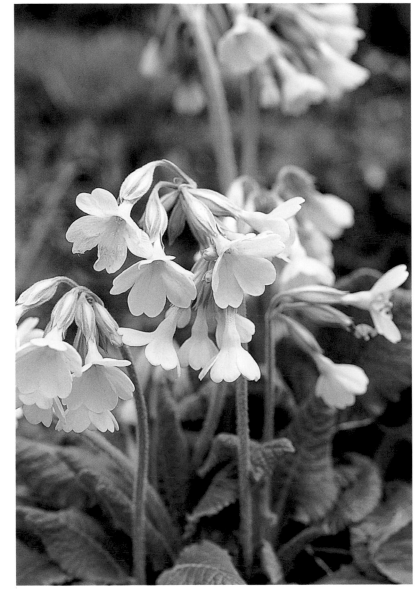

parts of the body). In general, however, reactions are mild, occurring within minutes of contact and subsiding again within just a few hours.

The majority of urticaria reactions are non-allergic and are due to irritant chemicals, such as preservatives (benzoic acid, sorbic acid, cinnamic acid), fragrances, medications applied to the skin, animal products, and plant products (including nettles and seaweed). Allergic (immunological) contact urticaria arises only if you place a protein to which you are sensitized on a damaged area of skin,

Primulas, although colourful additions to a garden or house-plant display with their attractive funnel-shaped flowers, can cause allergic skin rashes when handled.

such as a scrape or cut. When this happens, reactions can arise to proteins normally associated with food allergies, such as eggs, milk, nuts, fruit, seafood, and vegetables. Allergic reactions to preservatives, fragrances, and plant products are also possible. The most serious of these is latex allergy, which has the potential to cause widespread and very serious allergic responses (*see p. 23*).

INGESTED (FOOD) ALLERGIES

An adverse reaction to certain types of food can be either an abnormal response of the immune system to a food protein (a true food allergy), or it can be a chemical reaction to the food that does not involve the immune system (a food intolerance). Food intolerance is a more common condition than food allergy, although some instances of food allergy have been reported in approximately 1–2 percent of adults and in 5–7 percent of children.

Food allergy

True food allergy can give rise either to local symptoms in the stomach and gut, or to more generalized reactions. Contact with food to which you are allergic commonly causes a tingling of the lips and tongue followed by lip swelling (oral allergy syndrome). There may also be stomach cramping, bloating, and diarrhoea. In more severe examples, however, the following symptoms may occur:

- Tongue and throat swelling
- Facial flushing and swelling (angioedema)
- Difficulty in talking and breathing
- Fall in blood pressure causing dizziness and unsteadiness (anaphylaxis)

Certain, apparently unconnected, responses may also result from food allergies. For example, rhinitis (characterized by sneezing, a runny nose, and nasal congestion), asthma (difficulty in breathing, chest tightness, and wheezing), urticaria (itchy hives), eczema exacerbation (itchy skin rash), or arthralgia (painful joints).

Food intolerance

Non-allergic food intolerance may be due to the chemical properties of the food or to toxic reactions. Fish, such as mackerel and tuna, have high histamine levels when they start to spoil and these can cause flushing, low blood pressure, and hives – a reaction known as scombroid poisoning. And tyramine in red wine and cheese may cause a headache. Headache, along with flushing and gastrointestinal symptoms, can also be related to eating monosodium glutamate (MSG). Milk can cause abdominal pain and diarrhoea in infants. This is brought about by a deficiency in the baby's bowel of the enzyme lactase, which is necessary for the digestion of lactose, a sugar in milk. This deficiency can occur after a bout of infectious gastroenteritis.

Food additives and colourings may cause hives and make the symptoms of asthma and rhinitis far worse. Such reactions can occur to benzoates, salicylates, sulphites, and tartrazine. If your symptoms begin after eating foods containing preservatives or dyes, such as some cheeses, meat pies, sausages, preserved meat, dried fruit, and canned and bottled food, you should suspect the presence of these substances. Some preservatives are also sprayed on to salads to maintain freshness and can be present in alcoholic drinks and coloured fruit drinks (pop).

Oral allergy syndrome

This occurs in pollen-sensitive people when they eat foods containing a part of a protein structure that is the same as in pollen. The body mistakes the food for a pollen and initiates an allergic reaction. Reactions tend to be mild, confined to the lips and front of the throat, and disappear relatively rapidly. Ragweed- (*Ambrosia*) sensitive people may have oral symptoms after eating melons and bananas, while those sensitive to birch (*Betula*) pollen tend to react to raw potatoes, carrots, celery, apples, hazelnuts, and kiwi fruit.

THE PROBLEM FOODS

Just 8 foods cause about 90 percent of all food allergic reactions. They are milk, eggs, wheat, peanuts, soya (soy), tree nuts, fish, and shellfish. Milk is the most common cause of food allergy in children, most frequently giving rise to eczema, whereas peanuts, tree nuts, fish, and shellfish cause the most severe reactions. One-third of all medical emergencies for anaphylaxis (see pp. 22–3) are due to reactions to peanuts. Some people with peanut allergy are so sensitive that a reaction can occur after kissing someone who has eaten peanuts or merely smelling the nuts. Peanut allergy usually becomes apparent early in life – 55 percent of cases are known before the age of 3 years and 17 percent before the age of 1 year.

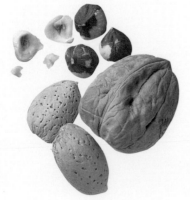

Atopic eczema

Otherwise known as atopic dermatitis, atopic eczema is the commonest form of allergy suffered by small infants. This disease is generally brought about due to a food allergy to dairy (milk) products or to eggs (generally egg white). Symptoms commonly include:

● Red areas with tiny bumps (papules)
● Blisters that weep
● Scaly skin

In infants, eczema often affects all of the body. As the baby grows and starts to toddle, the pattern of distribution changes, and becomes commonest in the bend of the elbows, at the back of the knees, and over the inside of the wrists. In the most severe cases, atopic eczema can affect any part of the body and cause a distressing, angry inflammation of the skin. The damage to the skin caused by this disease makes the child more susceptible to other environmental allergens, such as those associated with house-dust mites (see *pp. 36–7*). Two-thirds of children "outgrow" their food allergy by their fourth or fifth year. A child with a food-related allergy does, however, have an increased likelihood of developing asthma and rhinitis.

Coeliac disease

This condition results from a sensitivity to gluten, rather than being an allergy. Gluten is a protein found in cereals such as wheat, barley, oats, and rye. In susceptible individuals, eating gluten produces such symptoms as:

● An uncomfortable bloated feeling
● Wind and diarrhoea
● Malabsorption of food

Children with this disease do not grow as well as their peers, while in adults the malabsorption of food leads to weight loss. Since gluten-containing foods are so much a part of our everyday diet, a stringent programme of avoidance is necessary to avoid chronic ill-health. Gluten-avoidance does, however, result in the complete resolution of all symptoms.

SAFE ENTERTAINING

● Attending parties can be a problem for food-allergy sufferers as the content and preparation of the food is outside their control.
● Should a guest bring his or her own food to your party, or decline to eat the food provided, don't be offended – treat their concerns with sympathy.

● Eating nut-containing products can be life-threatening for nut-sensitive individuals, so keep nut products separate from other foods to avoid any chance of contamination.
● Pollen sufferers may experience a tingling and swelling of their lips when eating party foods such as apple, melon, celery, and cherry.

● Some colourings found in fruit juice or the preservatives contained in wine can induce wheezy episodes in asthma sufferers.
● Tobacco-smoke pollution at parties. If many of the guests are smoking, it can lead to the onset of symptoms for individuals with asthma, rhinitis, and conjunctivitis.

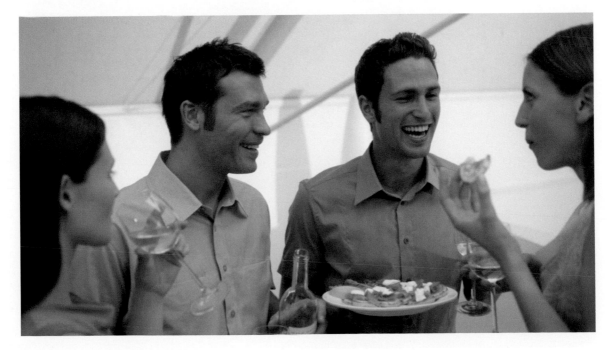

ANAPHYLAXIS

Symptoms of anaphylaxis may occur after eating certain foods; following an insect sting, such as that from a bee or wasp (yellow jacket); or an allergen contact (latex allergy, see *opposite*). In a sensitized person, the onset of anaphylaxis is characterized by a range of symptoms, although not necessarily all of the following will occur:

- Sense of foreboding, fear, and apprehension
- Flushing of the face, swelling of the lips, mouth, eyes, or tongue
- Generalized itching and the appearance of hives
- Tightness in the mouth, chest, or throat
- Difficulty experienced in breathing or swallowing, associated with drooling, wheezing, choking, and coughing
- Running nose
- Vomiting, nausea, diarrhoea, and stomach pains
- Dizziness, unsteadiness, sudden fatigue, rapid heartbeat, and chills
- Pallor, loss of consciousness, coma, and death

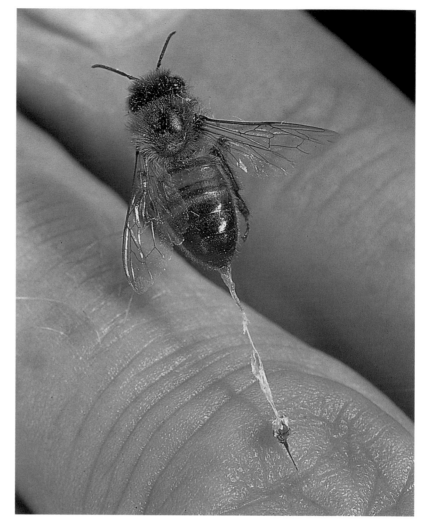

Stings from wasps (family Vespidae) or bees (family Apoidea) may precipitate a severe reaction, known as anaphylaxis, in some sensitized individuals.

The most serious allergic reactions occur to foods, such as fish, tree nuts crustaceans, and peanuts (see pp. 20–1), as well as to products that contain latex. While most of these problem foods are relatively easy to avoid, this is not necessarily the case with the groundnut, or peanut (*Arachia hypogea*), which is found in a surprisingly wide range of processed foods. The peanut is a member of the plant family Leguminosae, a family of plants that also includes beans, soya (soy) beans, kidney beans, peas, and lupins.

Peanut allergy

Of all the everyday foods, peanuts are the most problematic, and allergic reactions to them are often acute and severe. Such reactions can be fatal, and peanut allergy is the commonest cause of food-related allergy and anaphylaxis. In some parts of the

---

PEANUTS – HOW MUCH IS TOO MUCH?

The average protein content of a single peanut is 161mg, while approximately 50mg is all that is needed to cause a reaction in peanut-sensitive people – although some individuals are very much more sensitive. Since peanut allergy is for life, individuals who know that they react have to be extremely careful with their foods, and if they have any doubt they should avoid that food altogether. Although the peanut is of the same family as peas and beans, peanut-sensitive people do not tend to respond badly to these vegetables, but they may to tree nuts.

world, the average person consumes about 5kg/11lb of peanut products each year in the form of peanut butter, sweets (candy), baked goods, and table nuts. In those cultures, 80 percent of children have been exposed to peanut products by their first birthday and 100 percent by their second. Since peanut products are in a large range of processed foods, allergic reactions can occur on the first exposure to an actual nut, indicating that prior sensitization has already taken place, perhaps without individuals even realizing it. Some infant milk formulas used to contain peanut products, and peanut allergens are secreted in breast milk. Sensitization may even occur in infants as a result of mothers eating peanut-containing products when pregnant.

Peanut and other nut products may be encountered at any meal – in breakfast cereals, dried fruit and nut mixes, chilli and spaghetti sauces, gravies, oriental cooking, pastries, sweets (candies), ice creams, desserts, and garnishes. Removing the visible traces of nuts from food does not remove all traces of the offending protein.

In addition, it is possible for food contamination to occur through using utensils that have previously been in contact with peanuts. Concern also exists regarding protein contamination of peanut-oil preparations used in cooking. Such oils, also known in some countries as groundnut oil or arachis oil, may be sold simply as "vegetable oil".

Refined peanut oil does not contain peanut protein (the component to which individuals become sensitized), but if that oil is used to cook a product containing peanuts and is then reused, any other food cooked in it may become contaminated. The reuse of vegetable oils is widespread in homes, fast-food outlets, and in some restaurants.

Latex allergy

Natural rubber latex is a processed plant product derived almost exclusively from the tree *Hevea brasiliensis*, found in Africa and South East Asia. Natural rubber latex should not be confused with butyl- or petroleum-based synthetic rubbers. Latex is found in:

- Medical supplies, including disposable gloves, airway and intravenous tubing, catheters, and syringes
- Condoms
- Erasers (rubbers)
- Balloons
- Athletic shoe soles
- Automobile tyres
- Elasticated underwear, leg and waist bands
- Children's toys
- Dummies and infant pacifiers

Latex allergy occurs, for the most part, in well-defined groups, such as health-care and rubber-industry workers, and in children with bladder problems requiring permanent catheterization.

In latex-sensitive people, the presence of the weeping fig (*Ficus benjamina*) can cause asthma and other allergic reactions. This is because there is a cross-sensitivity between *Ficus benjamina* and *Hevea brasiliensis*. The weeping fig is a common ornamental plant in homes and offices, and the significance of its presence may not be fully appreciated. Latex-allergy sufferers may also react to such common foods as bananas, avocados, papaya, peaches, nectarines, and chestnuts, due to cross-sensitivity.

MEDICAL-ALERT JEWELLERY

A number of manufacturers produce medical bracelets and pendants that are intended to be worn permanently by people who are at risk from particularly severe medical conditions of the type that can suddenly overwhelm the sufferer. These "jewellery" items contain important medical details or a contact number to be used in case of an emergency.

Such jewellery is particularly useful for anaphylaxis patients as well as sufferers from severe asthma, especially a form termed "brittle asthma", whose condition can deteriorate into a life-threatening state very rapidly.

The largest manufacturer of medical-alert jewellery is MedicAlert, an internationally registered charity with affiliates in 22 countries and with more than 4 million wearers.

The MedicAlert bracelet carries an internationally recognized medical symbol and is engraved with the medical condition that the wearer suffers from, a personal identification number, and the organization's 24-hour emergency telephone number.

A telephone call made from anywhere in the world puts a medical professional through to a control room where the patient's computerized medical records are held on file. MedicAlert is a non-profit-making organization.

Other alert bracelets, such as the SOS Talisman (available in the UK), have a disc that unscrews and contains medical information that can be read on the spot in case of an emergency. This capsule is heat- and water-resistant and so the information is protected at all times.

Contributory Factors

The most commonly encountered allergens found within the average home are those to do with house-dust mites, cockroaches, and domestic pets (see pp. 36–7, 38–9, and 40–1). Pollen and mould allergens, although a widespread problem within the general population, normally represent only a minor component of the total allergen load found within the home. This is because, in most circumstances, you encounter these allergens only when you are outside.

Mould spores, pollen, and other allergens

Fungal growth – or, more to the point, the generation of the mould spores it produces (see pp. 42–3) – is a significant potential problem in homes where there is persistent dampness (see p. 136). Dampness in the home can be caused by a variety of factors, including the building's location and orientation, the lack of an adequate damp-proof course, a damaged roof, clogged guttering leading to rainwater overflow running down outside walls, ill-fitting or cracked downpipes (downspouts), or loose or badly maintained window frames. Apart from these causes of excess moisture, you could also have a ventilation problem (see pp. 50–7) giving rise to internal condensation, which is usually more pronounced on the inner surfaces of external walls.

As well as the generation of mould spores, dampness in the home is also associated with increased levels of house-dust mites and also with cock-roach infestation. All of these allergens have been linked with both the development and persistence of diseases such as asthma, rhinitis, and conjunctivitis and, to a lesser extent, to eczema as well.

In some homes, pollen can be a real problem for allergy sufferers (see pp. 28–31). For anybody acutely allergic to pollen, a single vase of cut flowers could be enough to trigger a reaction (see below). And the vogue in some parts of the world for adding conservatories (garden rooms) to existing homes, and then filling them with exotic plant species, can considerably increase the pollen count inside, especially if the conservatory has been fully integrated with the living room, dining room, or kitchen by the removal of the intervening external walls.

The same potential problem arises in homes with flower-filled sun-rooms or enclosed balconies or verandas if they have been integrated with the rest of the house or the connecting doors are not kept closed.

Allergy disease control

The control of allergens in the home is largely based on you having an understanding of both the source and nature of the allergen-producing substances affecting your condition. Other factors within the home, such as foods, cleaning products, cosmetics, and combustion by-products, can also play their role in the symptoms you experience, but these could be acting as irritants rather than allergens. While not actually the cause of allergic-like reactions, these irritants certainly can play an exacerbating role in the course of your allergic disease, increasing the intensity of the symptoms you experience.

A garden room with mostly non-flowering plants is preferable for pollen-sensitive individuals. Be aware too that plants increase humidity and may harbour mould (see p. 59 and p. 111).

DEALING WITH CUT FLOWERS

Allergy suffers who are particularly susceptible to pollen usually learn to avoid having cut flowers in their homes. However, if you choose the flower types carefully, it is still possible to enjoy a colourful vase of flowers inside. In an open flower the pollen is carried on stamens arising from the middle of the bloom. If the stamens are carefully removed before the pollen ripens and disperses into the air you should have few problems. The stamens of some flowers are too small and numerous for this to be feasible; others, however, such as lilies, have relatively few, very prominent stamens. These can be removed in a matter of seconds by a non-allergic family member as each flower opens, and the offending pollen taken away outside the home.

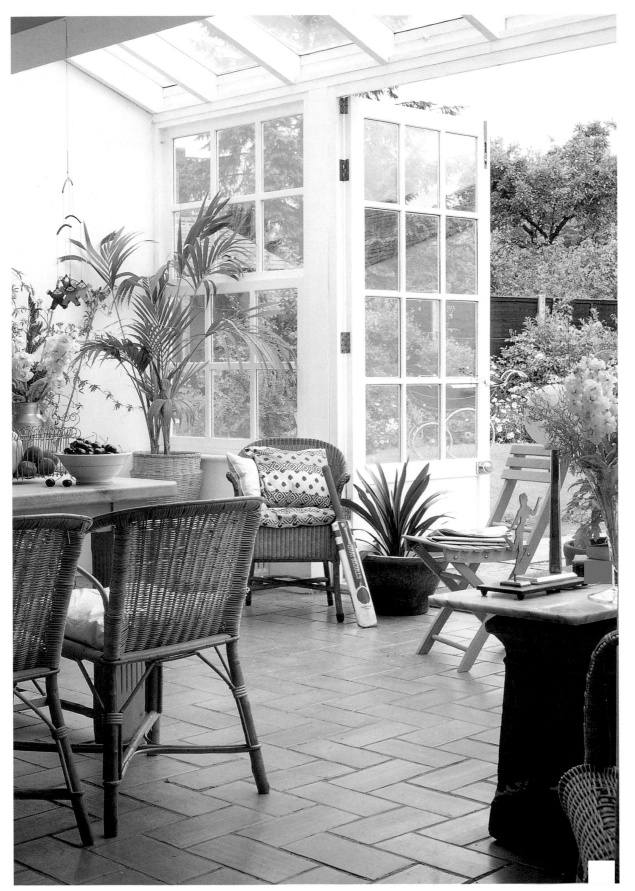

FAMILY AND LIFESTYLE FACTORS

Allergic problems tend to run in families, and the likelihood of a child developing an allergy is increased if one or both parents suffer from this problem. If both parents are allergic, the risk is 75 percent; if one parent is allergic, the risk is 50 percent. On average, between 10 and 20 percent of the population is allergic, although this is higher in certain age groups due to the increasing development of

Allergies such as asthma, hay fever, rhinitis, and eczema often run in families. This means that, unfortunately, more than one family member may be affected.

allergic problems in children. There is research evidence suggesting that the types of allergic disease the parents suffer from may influence the types of allergy their children develop. This is due to the inherited nature of the response to allergens and the body's response to the allergic reaction.

Early childhood infection

The immune system is still developing in early life and the stimulation of the immune system at this time by infections, such as respiratory infections with viruses or bacteria, or

even gastrointestinal infections, may help to direct the immune memory away from responding to environmental allergens and may, as a result, limit or even prevent the development of allergies.

Mild infections, such as those that are commonly experienced in childhood, may not always be sufficient to achieve this, but research is being conducted to identify if specific vaccinations to boost the immune response away from allergy and toward fighting infection may provide a preventative approach for the future.

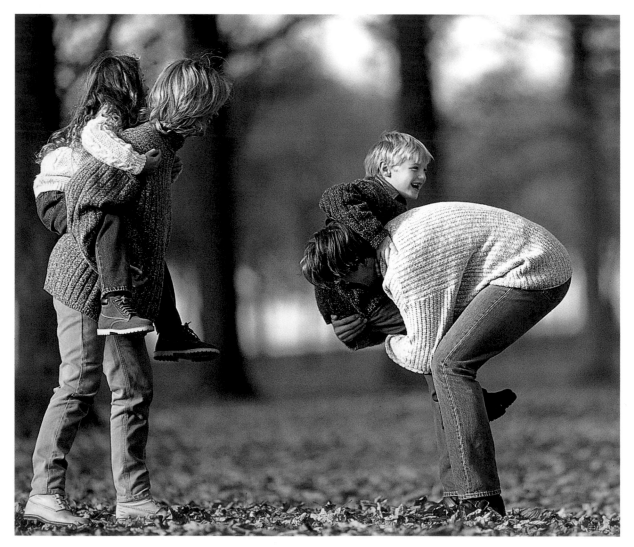

Asthma rates vary from country to country. In the UK, for example, one-third of 13–14 year olds are affected, while in the USA one-quarter of children in the same age group are affected.

Gender differences

Allergic problems are more common in boys than girls in childhood. Studies of children aged 13 show an increased likelihood of a heightened sensitivity to house-dust mite or cat allergen in boys compared with girls. This gender difference is less marked among adults, however, since males tend to "outgrow" their allergy.

Benefits of exercise

Some recent studies indicate that lack of exercise increases the likelihood of developing asthma. Whether this is due to the beneficial effects of exercise *per se*, or whether lack of exercise is an indicator of more time spent inside and greater exposure to household allergens is not clear. There does, however, appear to be advantages from exercise and the greater lung expansion associated with it.

Lifestyle factors

As well as there being geographical variations in the exposure to allergens, there are also regional and cultural differences in the likelihood of allergic diseases developing. For example,

DID YOU KNOW?

The prevalence of allergies is less common in younger children in large families than in their older brothers or sisters. The risk is almost half in the third or subsequent child compared with the risk of allergy in the firstborn. The reason for this is unknown, but one suggestion is that coughs and colds caught in early childhood from older siblings provide some protection from allergies.

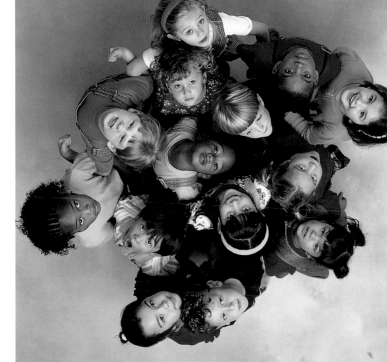

Prevalence of allergic disease in children

Parental allergy	Asthma	Hay fever	Eczema
Asthma	39%	0%	2%
Hay fever	3%	15%	5%
Eczema	2%	0%	10%

there is a lower incidence of allergic diseases in communities where a lot of natural and fresh foods are eaten, compared with communities, often more affluent ones, that are more reliant on processed foods. This may have something to do with the high level of anti-oxidants in natural, fresh food, including vegetables and fruit, and the high levels of preservatives and additives that are present in pre-prepared foods.

There is no doubt that the incidence of allergy is an increasing problem in societies that have an affluent lifestyle. Studies conducted in Africa on individuals from the same tribes (and, therefore, the same genetic backgrounds) identify higher incidences of asthma in urban as opposed to rural environments and in higher rather than lower social classes in the urban environment. Other research studies have shown that when immigrants move from a country with a basic standard of living to a more affluent society, they become more prone to asthma.

Factors associated with affluence that lead to the increase in asthma and in allergy are being studied, but the focus is on diet and lifestyle.

POLLEN

For many people, an allergy to pollen makes the spring, summer and/or autumn (fall) months a misery, confining them inside their homes with the windows and doors firmly shut. Although we think of brightly coloured garden plants as being the main pollen-producing culprits, many of the pollens produced by these flowers and flowering shrubs are too large for wind dispersal and do not, therefore, give rise to problems, unless you come very close to them. In fact, the major group of pollen sources associated with asthma, rhinitis, and conjunctivitis are tree, grass, and weed pollens.

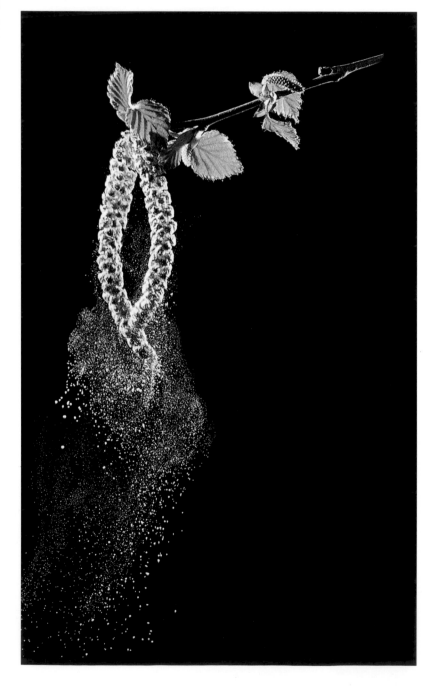

Some tree species, such as the birch (Betula) shown here, produce prolific amounts of pollen from laden catkins. Once ripe, the slightest breeze disperses the pollen far and wide.

Tree pollens

Trees are the first pollen producers of the year, releasing their showers of golden dust from the late winter and early spring through to the early summer. In Europe and the USA, depending on the distribution of species, the following trees may be associated with pollen allergy:

- *Acer* (Box elder)
- *Acer* (Maple)
- *Acer* (Sycamore)
- *Alnus* (Alder)
- *Betula* (Birch)
- *Carya* (Hickory)
- *Castanea* (Chestnut)
- *Cedrus* (Cedar)
- *Corylus* (Hazel)
- *Cupressus* (Cyprus)
- *Fraxinus* (Ash)
- *Juglans* (Walnut)
- *Olea* (Olive)
- *Populus* (Poplar)
- *Quercus* (Oak)
- *Salix* (Willow)
- *Ulmus* (Elm)

The pollination of trees depends on the ambient temperature and hours of sunlight, and since these factors are variable from year to year, so, too, is the amount of pollen produced. Typically, however, the pollen season for each tree species lasts about three or four weeks.

Grass pollens

Pollens that are produced by grass are generally more common than tree pollens, and grass pollinosis (the technical name for hay fever) affects a larger percentage of the population than tree pollinosis. The grass family (Poaceae) is extremely large, with more than 10,000 species worldwide. About 1,000 of these are distributed throughout the USA and only 400 in Europe. The grasses of lowland meadows tend to produce more pollen than those of poor soils. Grass pollens are too large to enter the lower airways, and so they are more often the cause of nose and eye problems rather than asthma. The common grasses that are associated with hay fever are:

- *Alopecurus* (Foxtail)
- *Anthoxanthum* (Vernal)
- *Arrhenatherum* (Oat grass)
- *Cornus* (Dogstail)
- *Festuca* (Fescue)
- *Lolium* (Rye)
- *Phleum* (Timothy)
- *Poa* (Meadow)

Grass pollens can be detected high up in the atmosphere and several kilometres out to sea and so are widely dispersed. As a result, local efforts to control levels are generally futile. Hay fever still occurs in cities even though areas of grassland are far fewer than in rural areas.

In cities, depending on the prevailing wind conditions and local geography, hay-fever attacks tend to peak one or two days after release of the pollens takes place in the countryside. Interestingly, the heat generated by cities keeps pollens airborne, so that ground-level measures of pollens are lower than in the country. However, this is not all good news, since the interaction of the pollens with city pollution leads to symptoms occurring at relatively low allergen levels.

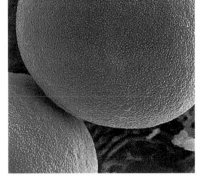

A high-power electron micrograph image allows tiny grass pollen grains to be seen in detail. Grass pollen is one of the culprits for hay fever.

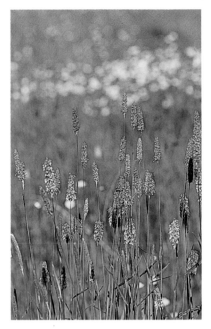

A meadow of Timothy grass (Phleum pratense) looks attractive in the summer, but it is not for those suffering with the symptoms of hay fever.

Weed pollens

Just when you think you are safe and can finally open your windows once again, having survived both the tree- and grass-pollen seasons, next it is the turn of the numerous weed species to add their pollen load to the air you breathe in.

The plant with one of the longest periods of pollination is the common dock weed (*Rumex*). This perennial weed begins pollinating in the early summer and does not finish until the mid autumn (fall). The weeds that are associated with the most significant problems are:

- *Ambrosia* (Ragweed)
- *Artemesia* (Mugwort)
- *Parieteria* (Nettle)
- *Parieteria* (Wall pellitory)
- *Plantago* (Plantain)
- *Rumex* (Dock)
- *Rumex* (Sorrel)

Ragweed (*Ambrosia*) is a prolific pollen producer and its pollen season in the northern hemisphere runs from August to November (or until the first frost,

REDUCING YOUR EXPOSURE TO POLLEN

- If you are buying trees for your garden, avoid species that produce the pollen likely to aggravate allergies (*see list opposite*).
- Whenever possible, limit your time outside during the pollen season, especially in the early morning and late evening, when pollen levels often peak.
- Keep windows in your home and car closed and keep cool with an air-conditioner.
- Don't hang your clothes outside to dry if there is a risk of pollen contamination.
- Pollen can be transported inside on people and pets.
- Check pollen count forecasts and daily levels before planning your day's activities.

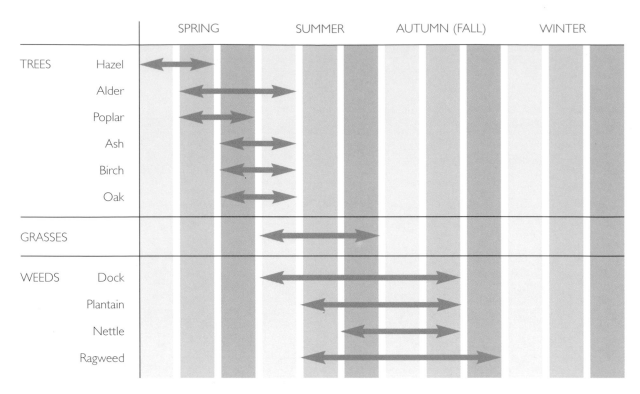

		SPRING	SUMMER	AUTUMN (FALL)	WINTER
TREES	Hazel	← →			
	Alder	← →			
	Poplar	← →			
	Ash	← →			
	Birch	← →			
	Oak	← →			
GRASSES			← →		
WEEDS	Dock		← →		
	Plantain		← →		
	Nettle		← →		
	Ragweed		← →		

whichever is sooner), and levels peak in mid September in many areas. Each plant produces about a billion pollen grains in a season and these have been detected 600 km/370 miles out at sea. Studies have shown that ragweed pollen is a very powerful allergen, with fewer grains needed to produce a hay-fever attack than with other allergens. Another significant plant is the wall pellitory, which also produces large amounts of a highly potent pollen.

A calendar of pollen prevalence starting in early spring – each band represents one month. There will be local variations depending on specific climate conditions.

Thunderstorm asthma

There are worldwide reports of severe asthma attacks occurring in association with thunderstorms during the hay-fever season. These attacks happen in individuals who suffer from hay fever but who do not usually experience asthma. It has been shown that grass pollens rupture in the high humidity preceding a storm, releasing large numbers of starch granules containing allergen. While pollen grains themselves are too large to be inhaled into the airways, these starch particles, either alone or bound to airborne particulates (such as diesel exhaust carbon particles), can readily be inhaled into the airways and induce an allergic reaction leading to asthma.

On occasions when "thunderstorm asthma" has occurred, pollen counts have been high and the high humidity has led to a great increase in starch granules containing allergen within the air. Sufferers need to be aware and stay inside if the weather forecast is bad.

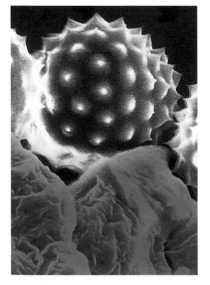

A high-power electron micrograph of a grain of pollen from a ragweed plant (Ambrosia). The colour seen here is not natural, but is added during the imaging process.

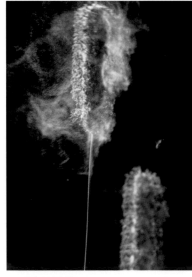

Looking like clouds of extremely fine dust, huge numbers of grass pollen grains are liberated and dispersed far and wide by the action of the wind.

THE EFFECTS OF WEATHER

In summer, pollen counts are high on sunny days due to flower pollination in the warm weather. Although peak levels occur early morning and late evening, high levels may be present throughout the day. Higher levels of pollen are more evident in rural than urban environments, but despite the lack of grassland, wind dispersal ensures the presence of pollen even in cities. Pollen counts tend to be much lower on rainy days, as the rain washes the pollen out of the air. However, it has been known that the number of hay-fever sufferers in congested cities seeking medical help for asthma increases after a thunderstorm. This is because the high humidity that often occurs before such a storm causes pollen grains to burst, each releasing hundreds of small starch particles. These particles, carrying one of the major grass allergens, become stuck to carbon diesel particles in polluted air. This combination is easily inhaled deep into the lungs, where it can trigger asthma attacks in hay-fever sufferers.

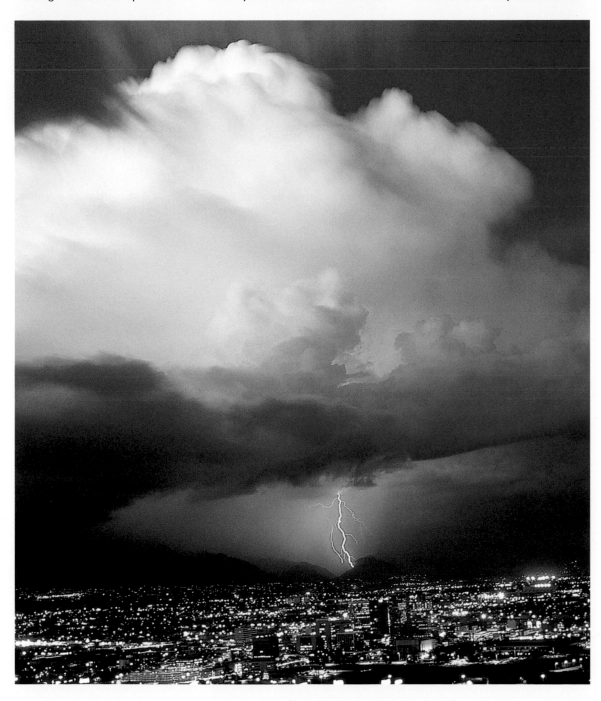

EXTERNAL AIR POLLUTION

The major outdoor air pollutants that allergy sufferers have to contend with are derived from burning fossil fuels – in particular, sulphur dioxide (SO_2), particulate matter (pm), nitrogen dioxide (NO_2), carbon monoxide (CO), acid aerosols, and ozone (O_3). Ozone is a secondary pollutant, and it is created when sunlight reacts with vehicle exhaust products (NO_2) in the presence of hydrocarbons. Ozone is, therefore, termed a photochemical pollutant. The importance of road traffic as a source of air pollutants, relative to other common sources, for a typical industrial country is illustrated in the table on the right.

The levels of outdoor air pollutants you are exposed to will depend on a number of factors, including local production, sunlight, and the prevailing

SOURCES OF PRINCIPAL OUTDOOR AIR POLLUTANTS

(percentage of total emissions)

SOURCE	SO_2	pm	NO_2	CO
Road transport				
Countrywide	2	47	51	90
City	22	96	76	99
Electricity generation	69	5	25	1
Other industrial pollution	21	4	12	2
Domestic (such as heating)	3	28	3	4
Other sources	4	15	8	3

winds. A high-pressure weather system, which is characterized by fine, hot weather with clear skies and little or no wind, will increase the likelihood of pollution-laden fog, or "smog".

External pollutants and allergies

The ever-increasing number of people suffering with allergies inevitably introduces the suspicion that pollution is responsible for these diseases. While the incidence of allergy has increased, air pollution, particularly that from sulphur-containing fossil fuels, has in fact decreased.

A study made after the reunification of Germany reported that there were higher levels of SO_2, NO_2, and particulate matter in Leipzig (old East Germany) compared with Munich (old West Germany). However, the much higher incidences of atopy (see p. 13) and allergic disease in Munich suggest that exposure to these outdoor pollutants does not increase the risk of allergy. Respiratory infections are, however, certainly increased by exposure to high levels of these pollutants, as are incidences of bronchitis.

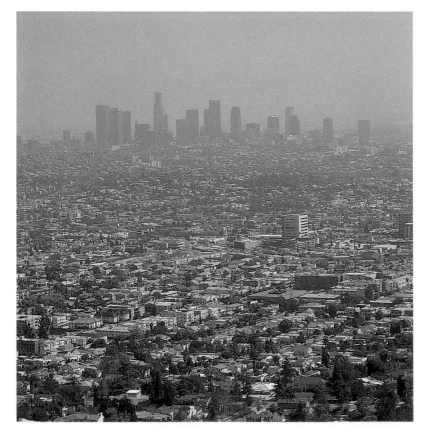

High levels of sunlight during the hot summer months combined with a lack of wind dispersion can result in thick smogs wherever traffic-exhaust pollution is a problem.

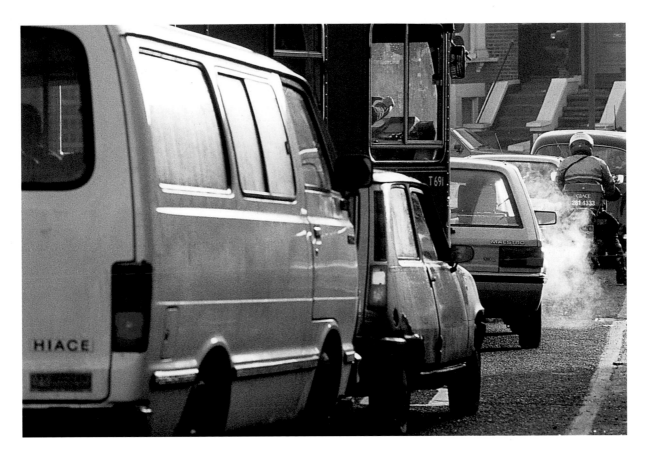

At road level, the exposure to the pollutant NO$_2$ (nitrogen dioxide) directly relates to the density of vehicular traffic.

Exposure to SO$_2$, NO$_2$, and ozone have all been shown to worsen asthma and rhinitis as well as contributing to conjunctival disease.

Allergen-pollution interactions

The worsening of asthma due to outdoor pollutants may occur for a number of reasons. For example, many of these pollutants are irritants, and so exposure to SO$_2$ and NO$_2$ may induce an acute narrowing of the airway. Associated with this is breathing difficulty, while exposure to ozone causes coughing and an inability to breathe deeply, which again leads to the sensation of breathlessness.

When you breathe through your nose, a process of absorption removes SO$_2$, and this helps to protect the lower airways. However, in individuals with allergic rhinitis, a symptom of which is a blocked nose, this crucial protection is lost, and when you breathe through your mouth, the SO$_2$ goes straight to the lower airways where it worsens the asthmatic condition. Similarly, when taking physical exercise you tend to breathe more through the mouth than nose. This means that jogging or cycling in polluted air, for example, will have a greater effect in worsening asthma than either the exercise or the pollution by itself.

Common external pollutants may also worsen any airway inflammation you already have, leading directly to a prolonged worsening of the asthma and a tendency to experience more severe attacks. This effect is most noticeable with ozone, where there is a 24-hour time delay between peak exposure and the worsening of your underlying condition.

EVERYDAY POLLUTANTS

Whether you live in country, town, or city, the air you breathe contains varying levels of pollutants.

SO$_2$ Sulphur dioxide is a colourless gas that readily dissolves in water. It reacts with water to generate sulphuric acid (H$_2$SO$_4$), which then falls as acid rain. Levels of SO$_2$ in the air are decreasing in areas where coal burning has decreased.

NO$_2$ Nitrogen dioxide is a strong oxidant. It is generated naturally by bacteria, volcanic action, and by lightning – but these sources result in only low background levels. The high levels in cities are concentrated at road level and correlate with the density of traffic.

O$_3$ Ozone is another powerful oxidizing agent, generated by the action of sunlight on traffic exhaust products.

HOUSEHOLD AIR POLLUTION

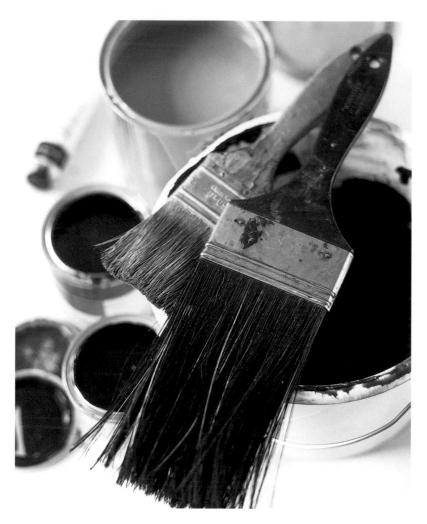

Home decorating with paints and varnishes give off fumes that may worsen allergic conditions. If at all possible, sensitive individuals should not be exposed to them.

include gas cookers (ranges), portable gas heaters, and wood-burning fireplaces, which all give off nitrogen dioxide. Sulphur dioxide, another problem indoor gas, comes from burning coal in open fires or from oil and paraffin heaters. Additionally, within the typical home environment are volatile organic compounds (VOCs), such as formaldehyde, which may be associated with respiratory problems (runny or blocked nose, coughs, and wheezing) and itchy skin.

Volatile organic compounds (VOCs)

These compounds are a group of chemicals based on the carbon atom (organic) that evaporate rapidly (volatile). There are many chemicals that fall into the VOC category, and in general they act as irritants – although a small percentage of allergy sufferers develop a specific immune response to VOCs, especially formaldehyde. Some VOCs occur naturally, such as when an orange is cut, while others are synthetic and are contained in

Most people spend more than 75 percent of their time inside, so their exposure to many common air pollutants is determined by the level of these substances found inside rather than outside. Air quality in a building will vary widely from one building to another depending on a variety of factors, including the production of chemicals and gases emitted from heating devices, internal fittings, and structural components. Another important factor in determining the level of air pollution inside is the rate of removal of these substances, which depends on how well your home is ventilated (*see pp. 52–7*).

The predominant pollutants, in general, act as irritants but they can also exaggerate allergic reactions to indoor allergens and make symptoms worse. The sources of these pollutants

AVOIDING POLLUTANTS IN THE HOME

- Do not allow tobacco smoking in the home.
- Maintain good air ventilation (*see pp. 54–7*)
- Consider potential sources of VOCs and decide to use alternative products if they are readily available.
- Carry out do-it-yourself jobs or hobby activities involving glues,

paints, varnishes, and solvents in well-ventilated areas or in a well-ventilated shed separate from the main house.
- Consider alternative cooking and heating methods to those associated with SO_2, NO_2, or VOC generation if anybody in your home is experiencing adverse reactions.

manufactured products, some common examples of which are listed here:

- Glues and solvents
- Board-based furniture
- Cleaning products
- Insulation material
- New carpets and some flooring
- Aerosol products
- Air fresheners
- Dry-cleaned garments
- Some synthetic fabrics
- Wood preservatives
- Paints – especially some gloss types

Passive smoking

Inhalation of second hand smoke fumes (passive smoking) is harmful to young children because it increases both their risk of developing a respiratory infection and their risk of developing an allergic tendency. It also potentially predisposes them to the development of asthma.

In addition, the presence of tobacco smoke pollutants within the air act as irritants to worsen pre-existing allergic diseases. Thus, going into a smoky environment will make the eyes sore and water in individuals with conjunctivitis, worsen nasal blockage in those with rhinitis, and may induce chest tightness, wheeze, and cough in people with asthma.

Thus, for children living with parents who smoke, the constant exposure to airborne tobacco pollution will worsen the children's allergic conditions, whether this is asthma, rhinitis, or conjunctivitis, and thus stronger maintenance treatment will be necessary than in a non-smoking home.

If you are painting or varnishing in a confined space, keep the area well ventilated or wear a protective mask with an activated carbon filter to absorb the fumes.

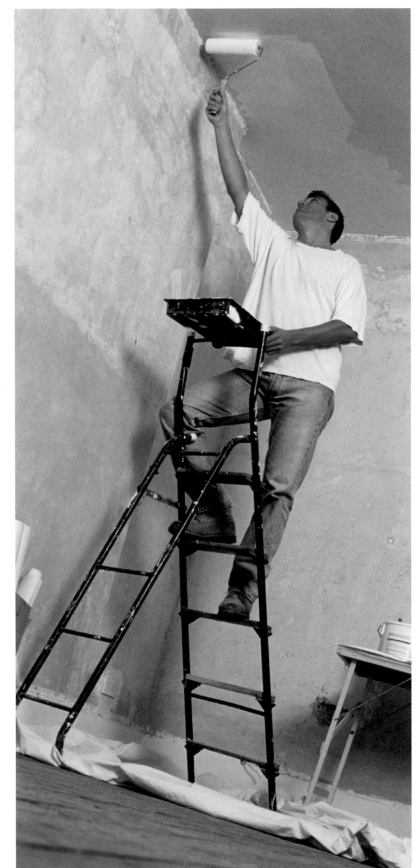

HOUSE-DUST MITES

Lurking unnoticed, too small to be seen without the aid of a microscope, the house-dust mite is the natural scavenger within our homes.

Why are mites a problem?

House-dust mites are members of the arachnid family — a family that includes spiders, chiggers, and ticks. Like spiders, they have eight legs, but the mites themselves are sightless and completely harmless, since they do not bite, sting, or transmit diseases of any description. Their natural diet consists of shed human skin scales, plant fibres, house dust, fungal spores, pollen grains, and insect scales.

In themselves, they pose absolutely no problems to people, unless, that is, you are one of the many thousands who have an allergic reaction to the proteins contained in their fecal droppings.

Huge populations of these mites exist in our homes, particularly within the fibres of bedding, carpeting, and upholstered furniture. To give you some

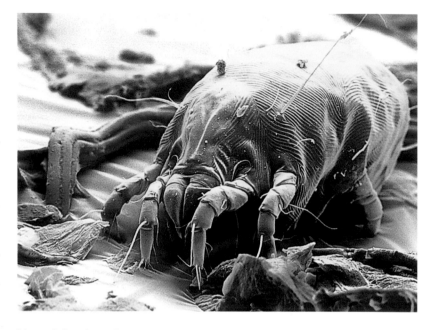

idea of the size of creature you are dealing with, up to 1,000 individual mites can be counted in just 1 gram of dust (and there are approximately 28 grams in an ounce). This means that the average bed contains more than 10,000 dust mites and perhaps in excess of two million fecal pellets.

The usual route for these fecal pellets to enter the body is through contact with the mucous surfaces of

Seen here magnified many thousands of times, the house-dust mite (Dermatophagoides pteronissius) feeds on the organic components contained in dust.

the nose, the lining of the eyes, or the lining in the airways of the lungs. Being so tiny, once the pellets have been disturbed by such everyday actions as sitting on a bed or an upholstered chair, couch, or sofa, they remain airborne for at least 30 minutes before settling once more. These pellets also tend to settle at other sites within your home, such as in the fibres of curtains, drapes, or carpets. Children playing on the floor, will therefore, be particularly at risk in carpeted homes.

House-dust mite biology

Just how many house-dust mites you have in your home depends not so much on how thoroughly you clean and dust, but rather on the indoor humidity and temperature.

House-dust mites do not drink to satisfy their thirst; instead they absorb

---

REDUCING YOUR EXPOSURE TO HOUSE-DUST MITES

- Cover mattress and bedding (duvet, pillows) with anti-mite barrier covers (see pp. 82–3).
- Wipe clean anti-mite barrier covers with a damp (not wet) cloth every time you change the bedlinen.
- Wash anti-mite covers every 6–12 months, according to the manufacturer's instructions.
- Remove soft toys from children's bed, especially at night. An exception is a favourite toy, which must be washed regularly or placed in the freezer for several

hours, to minimize build-up of house-dust mite (see p. 89).
- Avoid clutter on ledges where dust can accumulate.
- Remove carpeting (see pp. 62–4).
- Vacuum regularly (see pp. 74–5).
- Replace fabric-upholstered furniture with leather or vinyl if possible (see p. 70).
- Keep rooms ventilated (see pp. 54–7).
- Reduce humidity within the home (see p. 58).
- Install washable curtains or vertical blinds (see p. 65).

GEOGRAPHICAL DISTRIBUTION

The term "house-dust mite" is used to encompass about 10 different species of the Pyroglyphidae family of the arachnids. Out of this family, four are most frequently encountered and they are known by their Latin names: *Dermatophagoides pteronissius, Dermatophagoides farinae, Dermatophagoides microcerus,* and *Euroglyphus maynai.* The term *Dermatophagoides* literally translates as "skin-eating". The *D. pteronissus* and *E. maynai* mites are the most frequently encountered in Europe, while these and *D. farinae* are all equally common throughout North America. One further house-dust mite, *Blomia tropicalis,* is prevalent in tropical and semitropical areas and is, therefore, to be found in Florida, along the Gulf Coast, and in South American countries Venezuela and Brazil. Another group of mites, known as the "storage mites" (families Acaridae, Glycyphagidae, and Chortoglyphidae), also occur in house dust, but they are less prominent than those of the Pyroglyphidae family, which account for about 80–90 percent of the mites present in house dust.

water directly from the air through special glands in their skin. They grow best in a relative humidity of between 75 and 80 percent. Relative humidity is the percentage of the maximum possible amount of water vapour in the air – saturation, in other words – which, in turn, is dependent on the ambient temperature. Temperature is important because warmer air is capable of holding more moisture than is cooler air. If the relative humidity falls, there is simply not enough water vapour to allow the mites to thrive and reproduce.

One of the approaches in at least limiting the numbers of house-dust mite in your home is, therefore, to regulate the level of air humidity. This in itself cannot be a complete control, however, as mites have a protective mechanism to prevent excessive dehydration when the humidity falls.

Studies have shown that house-dust mites can maintain a water balance and survive at relative humidities of around 45 percent at 15°C/59°F; 55 percent at 25°C/77°F; and 65 percent at 30°C/86°F.

The other major factor, apart from air humidity, regulating the number of house-dust mites that your home is likely to be playing host to, is the ambient temperature. Mites cannot shiver or sweat in order to regulate their own body temperature, and so they are entirely dependent on the temperature of the surrounding air for their survival. The ideal temperature, as far as the mite is concerned, is about 25°C/77°F. Therefore, if you keep the temperature of your home below this level you will inhibit their numbers.

The body temperature of house-dust mites governs their metabolic rate. This means that both egg production and life expectancy decrease at low temperatures, which leads to a decline in the total number of mites. This is the reason why people whose dust-mite sensitivity results in asthma attacks often find relief in high-altitude environments, where both humidity and the ambient air temperatures are too low for the mite to survive.

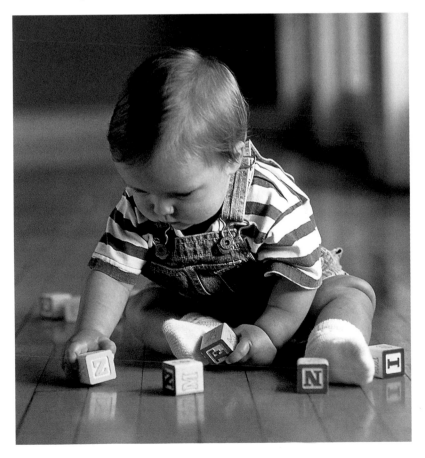

Because babies and young children spend so much of their time in close contact with the floor, removing carpets helps to reduce their exposure to house-dust mite allergen.

COCKROACHES

Cockroaches, which are also known as waterbugs, croton bugs, and palmetto bugs, are second only to house-dust mites as a cause of allergy in some countries. Although cockroaches are usually associated with the hotter, more humid regions of the world, they are also prevalent in more temperate countries where central heating is used to maintain a high temperature in the home during the colder winter months.

Cockroach infestation and allergy is a common problem in many countries, including the USA, Taiwan, Japan, Thailand, and Singapore, as well as throughout South America and in South Africa and Australia. In Europe, surveys suggest that about 5–10 percent of the population are cockroach-sensitive, making it far less of a concern than in the USA, where the figures suggest that 40–60 percent of the population have this problem.

Where are cockroaches found?

There are many different species of cockroach – about 50 in total – varying in size from about 2–5cm/ ¾–2in. Some species live mainly outdoors, entering into your home only to breed or to search for food.

These insects are usually found around kitchen sinks or draining boards, underneath or in cracks around cabinets and cupboards, inside cabinets (especially in the upper corners), behind drawers, around pipes or conduits (where they pass along a wall or go through it), behind windows or door frames, behind loose skirting boards or moulding strips, on the underside of tables or chairs, and in the bathroom. They are even sometimes found living in the back of radios or televisions.

The widely distributed German cockroach is generally to be found in kitchens and bathrooms, although these insects can also be present just about anywhere, whereas the other species generally prefer dark environments, such as those in garages, basements, and attics.

The cockroach is also a common inhabitant of sewers, and often after heavy rainfall you find that their numbers increase in basement areas.

Cockroaches are commonly found anywhere that food is available for them to eat, either in food-storage areas or around dustbins (garbage cans). Being aware of these potential sources of infestation is important when you are trying to restrict their movement into your home.

Cockroach biology

Water is the most important factor in determining cockroach survival. German cockroaches can survive for 42 days on just water alone but only

KNOW YOUR COCKROACH

Cockroaches are brown, black, or tan shiny insects that can fly. They secrete an oily liquid, which has an unpleasant odour, on to food and surfaces around the home. Excrement, in the form of pellets or an ink-like fluid, also contributes to this nauseating smell. Cockroaches hide in dark, sheltered places during the day and normally come out to feed only at night.

These insects (Order: *Orthoptera*) fall into the family Blattidae (derived from the Latin *blatta*, which means "flees from light"), and there are five types of cockroach that are commonly found in houses, although more than 50 species exist. The commonest species in the home is the German cockroach (*Blattella germanica*), which is about 2cm/ ¾in long. A single pair of

these insects can produce up to 30,000 offspring in just one year.

The cockroach has three life stages: egg, nymph, and adult. The eggs of cockroaches are deposited in a leathery case, which is generally glued in a hidden crack, with the exception of the German cockroach, which carries its capsule until the eggs are about to hatch. There are 38–40 eggs per case with the German cockroach, and less with other species (10–28 eggs).

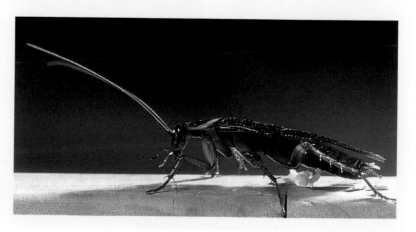

AVOIDING COCKROACH ALLERGENS

- Reduce sources of dampness in the home (see pp. 52–3).
- Maintain good air ventilation see pp. 54–7).
- Promptly dispose of all waste food and other waste matter in sealed bags or containers and keep the surrounding area clean.
- Keep food in sealed containers or inside the refrigerator.
- Don't leave plates and other crockery unwashed overnight to become cockroach feeding sites.
- Keep pet food in resealable containers and do not leave food and water out all the time.
- Vacuum regularly to remove food crumbs (see pp. 74–5).
- Seal entry sources into your home, such as those around

- pipework – an adult cockroach can squeeze through an opening only 1.6mm/¹⁄₁₆in wide.
- Keep rooms uncluttered. This provides the cockroach with fewer hiding places.
- Seal cracks and crevices in woodwork.
- Don't overwater your houseplants and so make moisture available.
- Inspect grocery bags for cockroaches before putting food away in cabinets.
- Use traps (see below).
- Consider using chemical controls – readily available as sprays, concentrates to be mixed with water, baits, and dusts – but always follow the manufacturers' instructions regarding safe usage.

12 days if the water supply is withdrawn, even if there is plenty of food to eat.

This accounts for the fact that you tend to see more cockroaches in the home during prolonged periods of drought, since it is then that the insects move inside looking for a reliable water supply.

Ensuring that there is no standing water anywhere readily available is, therefore, one of the main strategies that you can adopt to prevent cockroach infestations. Even what you might consider to be inconsequential amounts of water can be a lifeline for the cockroach, so make sure to wipe draining boards completely dry after washing up the dishes and basin surrounds after cleaning your teeth.

In apartment blocks and terraced housing, however, it is difficult to eliminate all suitable cockroach environments, no matter how careful you might be, since the potential for reinfestation from neighbouring properties is always a possibility.

Why are cockroaches a problem?

The source of cockroach allergen is less well defined than for the house-dust mite, but it is probable that digestive enzymes present in their fecal particles play an important role.

Although cockroach fecal particles are substantially larger and heavier than those of the house-dust mite, they could still become airborne, and so be available to be breathed in through the nose or mouth or enter the body through the eyes, if they become fragmented. It is also possible that dust particles could become coated with the insects' allergens and enter the body along with the inhaled dust particles. Some research has also suggested that the cockroach sexual pheromone-binding proteins, rather than the fecal droppings, may be the source of the secreted allergens.

In socially deprived, inner-city areas with poor housing, cockroach allergy has been found to be a major factor in those attending hospital emergency departments with severe asthma. Cockroach allergy can be tested for using a skin-prick test (see pp. 44–5).

Cockroaches can also act as disease carriers. They are known to carry human infections and food poisoning bacteria.

USING AND MAKING COCKROACH TRAPS

Sticky traps made specifically for cockroaches can be bought from hardware stores. You should place these inside in the most likely cockroach feeding or watering sites, such as near the waste container, under the sink, in food cabinets, under and behind the refrigerator, and in the bathroom. Sticky traps are not recommended for use outside because they generally do not hold the larger cockroach species found outside and they are not resistant to the elements. You can, however make your own, very effective, cockroach trap for the home with little effort:

- Take any empty jar that has a rounded lip and grease the inside upper surface with a thin film of petroleum jelly.

- Place a quarter slice of beer-soaked bread, or any other food, in the jar.
- Wrap the outside walls of the jar with paper towel to help the cockroaches climb to the top, so that they can then fall in.
- Place the jar against a wall to give the insects easy access to the bait, or otherwise place the jar as for the sticky traps.
- Outside, cover the jar with a domed shape of aluminium foil to prevent rain filling into the trap, but keep the side access open to admit the cockroaches.
- To kill the trapped cockroaches, pour dishwashing detergent into the jar and add hot water. Wash the jar and relay the trap every 2–3 days.

DOMESTIC PET ALLERGY

Domestic pets are an extremely common cause of allergies within the home. The worst offenders are cats and dogs, and contact with these animals can result in asthma, rhinitis, or conjunctivitis. Allergic reactions are also associated with birds, mice, rats, guinea-pigs, rabbits, and hamsters. Allergy problems with outdoor animals, such as geese, ducks, chickens, and horses, are also common.

The allergens themselves are found in the animal's skin flakes (dander), as well as in their hair, saliva, and urine, and they quickly become distributed throughout any home where pets live. Due to their sticky nature, these allergens can be transported on people's clothing, therefore ending up in rooms, or even other buildings, where animals have been excluded. This can be a real problem for allergy sufferers when they are visited by their pet-owning friends.

Cat allergy

The most common pet allergy is to cats, with up to 40 percent of asthma sufferers showing some degree of sensitivity. The major cat allergen is found in cat saliva and its sebaceous and lacrimal glands. During grooming, when the cat licks itself, this allergen is transferred on to the fur and, after it has dried, is shed into the air. This allergen is widely distributed, more so than mite allergen, as it is far smaller and can remain airborne for hours. When the cat is present in a room, however, the airborne allergen tends to increase by approximately fivefold. Since cat allergen particles are so small, they are easily inhaled, and people sensitized to the substance commonly experience symptoms soon after coming into contact with it, whether or not a cat is actually in the room. Castrated male cats produce between three and five times less allergen than uncastrated males.

Cat allergen readily sticks to carpeting, furnishings, and walls and is difficult to eradicate – levels can still be detected in dust for months after a cat has gone. Bear this in mind when moving house, and be prepared to wash down walls thoroughly and have all the carpets and curtains removed or professionally cleaned.

Dog allergy

Allergy to domestic dogs is less common than allergy to cats. The source of the allergen is the same,

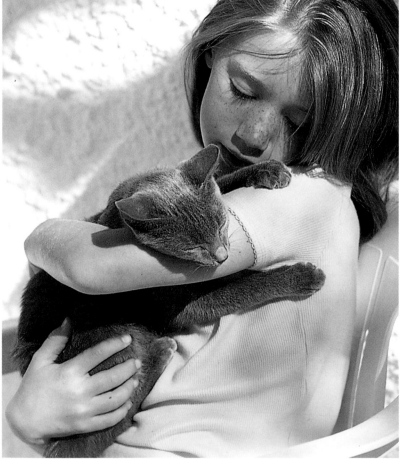

Although a difficult decision to have to make, household pets, especially the much-loved cat, may have to be banned from the homes of allergy sufferers.

however – dander, saliva, and urine – and studies have shown that dog allergen is present in more than half households sampled.

Since saliva is one of the most important sources of allergen, a dog's lick may set off a severe response. Some people report the onset of symptoms only after contact with specific breeds. There is no good evidence that different breeds have different allergens – but it could be that individual dogs vary in the amount of allergen that they generate.

Allergies to other pets

With household pets such as rabbits, rats, mice, hamsters, and guinea-pigs, the most important sources of allergen are saliva and urine. Rodents excrete protein in their urine, which dries and becomes airborne on dust particles, allowing its inhalation. Although hair and skin particles also carry allergen, these allergens are primarily derived from contamination with urine and saliva.

Horse and cow skin scales can be allergenic to those exposed to them, and horse allergen sticks readily to clothing and so is liable to be transported into the home. Birds carry allergy-provoking mites, moulds,

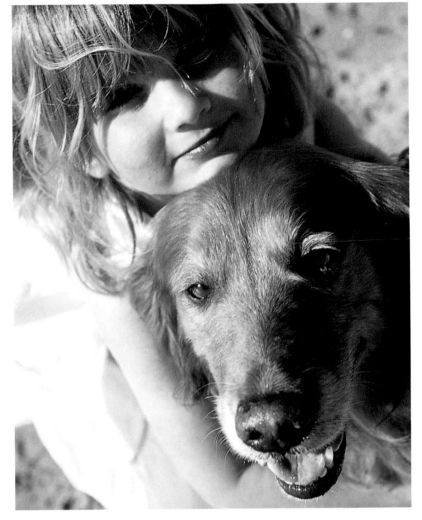

and pollens on their feathers. Budgerigar droppings contain a protein that becomes airborne and can induce a lung problem that is separate from the usual forms of

Dogs generally cause fewer and less severe allergic problems for people than do cats, but in some people a simple "dog lick" is enough to induce an allergic response.

allergy. This problem is insidious in its onset and leads to progressive breathlessness and cough.

Although fish are generally considered safe for people who are allergic to the more usual pets, sensitization to ants' eggs, a fish food, has been reported. Moulds may also grow in damp areas around or inside fish tanks, and the spores of this can be a cause of allergic reactions. Some fishkeepers have been known to develop skin rashes on their hands, but the offending substance involved could be an irritant rather than an allergen.

AVOIDING PET ALLERGENS IN THE HOME

- Ideally, you should remove all pets from the home.
- Keep pets outdoors if possible and, if not, keep them in well-ventilated parts of the house with hard flooring, such as in the kitchen.
- Do not allow pets in bedrooms or in the main living rooms.
- Wash cats and dogs frequently (at least once a week) to remove allergens from their fur or hair.
- Vacuum floors, bedding, and soft furnishing regularly with a high-

efficiency particulate air (HEPA) filter and use double-thickness vacuum cleaner bags to prevent the allergen leaking (see pp. 74–5).
- Install HEPA air filters (see p. 57) in bedrooms and living rooms.
- Remove carpeting and install linoleum/vinyl/wood flooring instead (see pp. 63–4).
- Clean upholstered chairs and couches or sofas weekly, or replace them with leather- or vinyl-covered furniture (see p. 70).

MOULD ALLERGY

As well as being commonly found outdoors, mould spores are also present inside the home, especially anywhere that is persistently damp and poorly ventilated (see p. 50).

Growing conditions

The water needed for the growth of the mould that produces the mould spores comes principally from rising damp, water penetration, leaking pipes, and high relative-humidity levels. High relative humidity is commonly brought about by a combination of inadequate ventilation and water vapour condensing on cold surfaces, such as windows in bathrooms and kitchens and the inside surfaces of external walls. Therefore, older houses, which often have inadequate heating and poor ventilation, are more prone to dampness than newer properties. Once moulds are established in the

house, they will also grow on items of fresh or stored food, as well as on other household goods such as books.

Types of mould

The commonest indoor moulds are those relating to the *Aspergillus* spp. and the *Penicillium* spp. which grow

---

CONTROLLING MOULD SPORES

- Check for signs of mould in showers or in dark, moist parts of your home where there is poor ventilation and an external wall.
- Clean showers, window sills, kitchens, basements, or other areas where moulds might grow with a bleach solution, and then treat them with a mould inhibitor.
- Provide good ventilation – for example, by installing an extractor (exhaust) fan – in the bathroom to reduce mould growth (see p. 55).
- Keep a bright light bulb burning in a closet if there is no heating to help dry it out.
- Clean guttering and downpipes regularly to prevent water penetrating from outside.
- Ensure that all window frames are properly sealed and replace any rotten frames or cracked boards.
- Repair any defects in your damp-proof course.
- Don't leave rotting food and fruit about the home.
- Remove all traces of food from surfaces inside the home.

---

well wherever the air reaches more than about 70 percent relative humidity. *Aspergillus niger* is dark brown and is chiefly responsible for the typical patches of black on persistently damp walls and skirtings.

To survive and grow, these moulds literally eat the paint or wallpaper, cotton, and other cellulose material. They also eat dust and any minute pieces of food material on walls. *Penicillium* is the mould used in the manufacture of "blue" cheeses. It is commonly found in stored fruit, and foods such as cheese and bread. (Note that this has nothing to do with allergy to the drug penicillin.)

Outdoor moulds can migrate into buildings, although usually at lower concentrations. However, if conditions are favourable – in other words, damp – they can greatly increase in number.

Carpeting provides a perfect reservoir for dust and spores, which can become airborne whenever they

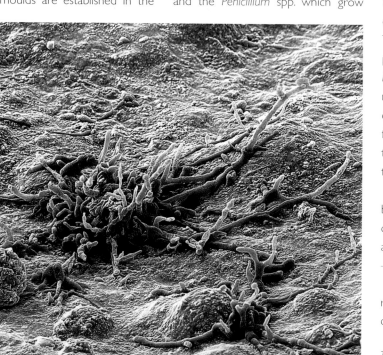

This strange looking alien landscape is, in fact, an electron-micrograph image of a common mould, showing mould hyphae, growing on the inside surface of a wall.

are disturbed. The concentrations of spores in the air depend largely on the level of activity in the home — larger concentrations typically occur if any building work or repairs are being carried out and when you are cleaning. Vacuum-cleaning carpets, for example, has been reported to increase considerably mould spore numbers in the air and, once airborne, they can float about waiting to be breathed in for at least an hour before settling back down.

Does air conditioning help or hinder?

In hot climates it is worth considering installing air conditioning (see pp. 58–9), since, as well as cooling the home, it reduces the amount of mould allergen in the air by filtering it out and reducing humidity. Air conditioning also has another benefit — it allows you to reduce the number of windows that you need to keep open, thus limiting the number of spores entering the home from the outside world.

These systems, however, need to be properly maintained to prevent condensation on the cooling coils from building up, and to remove any stagnant water from the system, both of which could encourage mould growth (such as Aspergillus and Penicillium). When mould does establish itself, its spores will then be dispersed freely around the building by the action of the air-conditioning system itself, and this effect has been associated with very high levels of fungal spores within homes.

Outdoor mould allergen exposure

Outside, the level of mould spores in the atmosphere will vary depending on the season. Levels typically range

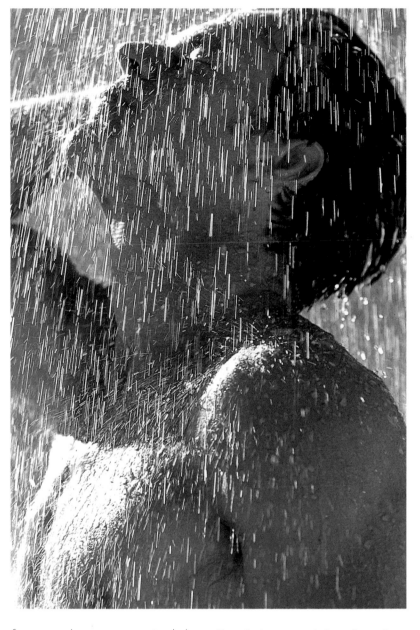

from very low spore counts during the cold winter months to high counts between late summer and early autumn (fall).

While local and regional variations are very usual, the commonest spores across a range of different environments are derived from Cladasporium and Alternaria species, which grow on rotting vegetation. Allergic reactions to mould spores are less common than those to grass pollen (see pp. 28–31), but when sensitization does occur in individuals, these allergens

Showering is an economical use of water, but you need to take care that mould growth does not occur in the shower cubicle or on the shower curtain or screen.

give rise to similar problems (see pp. 16–17), causing sneezing, a runny or blocked nose (rhinitis), and itchy, watery eyes (conjunctivitis).

Since mould-spore prevalence will be on the increase just as the grass-pollen season is coming to an end, sufferers with dual sensitivity will unfortunately experience a prolonged "hay-fever" season.

Diagnosis and Management

The diagnosis of an allergic disease has to be based on a careful medical history taken by a doctor, and you may have to be referred to a specialist. All your symptoms need to be described in detail before a doctor can determine whether or not you have an allergic disease and decide on a course of management.

The nature of any conditions that make the symptoms worse, or trigger factors, and the frequency and duration of your symptoms, are all important considerations. Not all problems, even though they may be similar to those produced by allergens, are, in fact, allergic in nature.

A tendency to house-dust mite allergy, one of the most common of all allergies, is suggested by several "yes" responses to questions such as, for young children:

● Does your baby sneeze when you lay him or her on the bed in the morning?
● Is your child often troubled with conjunctivitis and eczema?
● Did your toddler get a "cold" and cough when moved to the "big" bed, and has continued snuffling ever since?
● Do your children appear to contract a "cold" when they stay with relatives or friends?
● Have you had a positive skin test to mites?

And, for adults and older children:
● Do you sneeze, get itchy hands or face, or become breathless when making the bed and vacuuming?
● Do you sneeze or get a tight chest in the morning or after getting into bed at night ?
● Do you wake up at night with itchy eczema or a blocked or runny nose and are kept awake because of it?
● Do you get night asthma?
● Do you feel better when you are outside the home?
● Do your symptoms disappear on holiday (vacation) in a warm, dry climate, only to reappear soon after returning home?
● Do your symptoms become worse in the autumn (fall)?

The presence of an allergic tendency is suggested by a family history of allergic problems and can be tested for by checking whether or not you have an elevated immunoglobin E (IgE) response to specific allergens

Skin-prick tests

The most widely used allergy test is the skin-prick test (*see below and opposite*). This is based on the fact that IgE binds to special cells in the skin, called mast cells, and that when allergens come into contact with the IgE the mast cells release chemicals that produce an itchy reddening of the skin with a central bump. The size of the bump reflects the strength of the reaction. Many tests to different allergens can be carried out at once. Results are apparent after about 15 minutes.

Blood tests

A blood sample can be analyzed for specific IgE. The laboratory will check for single allergens as well as for

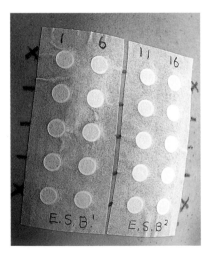

In a patch test, samples of different allergens are placed against the skin and left in place for two or three days before being inspected for a reaction.

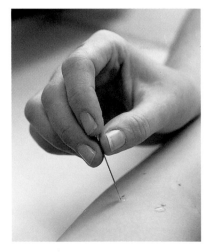

A skin-prick test is routinely carried out in order to test an individual's sensitivity to airborne and food allergens. A reaction is usually apparent within 15 minutes.

multiple allergens. The advantages of a blood test are that it is not influenced by drug treatment and can be given to people who have widespread skin diseases. The disadvantages, compared with skin-prick tests, are that blood tests are expensive, may not be as sensitive, and results are not instant.

Patch tests

A patch test is widely used in the diagnosis of contact allergies (*see opposite*). Several standard series of contact allergens are available. These are placed on the skin (often on the back), strapped in place, and left for between 48 and 72 hours before the skin is inspected. These tests can be undertaken only by an expert, since it is important to distinguish an allergic response from an "irritant response".

Treatments

Once the diagnosis of allergy has been made there are three main approaches to treatment, which all complement each other but which vary from condition to condition in their relative merits and relative importance. These treatments are allergen avoidance, drug treatment, and desensitizing therapy.

Allergen avoidance

The basis for all allergy treatments is allergen avoidance where possible; avoiding whatever it is that induces the response will hopefully lead to an improvement. This is clear in seasonal hay fever, since symptoms disappear once the pollen season is over. Similarly, clinics at high altitude, where conditions are unfavourable for the house-dust mite, have reported clear improvements in children and adults whose asthma is brought on by mites. Where occupational-allergic asthma is the problem, provided that the disease is recognized early enough, removing the sufferer from the offending environment leads to an improvement. In addition, allergic skin diseases, such as contact dermatitis, will improve once the offending agent is identified and avoided.

Therefore, the key to allergen avoidance is the correct diagnosis and identification of the inducing allergen. *The Allergen-free Home* section (*see pp. 48–128*) looks in detail at the different allergens in the various rooms of the home and identifies approaches to reducing your exposure to, or avoiding allergens within, the home environment.

Drug therapy

A range of drug therapies that suppress symptoms, or that suppress the inflammation resulting from your exposure to allergens, can be used to treat a variety of diseases, including asthma, rhinitis, conjunctivitis, urticaria, and eczema. But all of these therapies need to be discussed with your doctor, who may refer you to a specialist. These treatments do not cure the allergy and the allergic diseases often come back once the treatment has been discontinued. If taken regularly by people with daily symptoms, however, they do provide very effective relief.

There are certain classes of drug that are common to several of the conditions, the most commonly used being antihistamines.

Antihistamines This class of drug can be used in the eye (drops), in the nose (spray), or taken orally (tablet or liquid), and it is one of the first lines of treatment for mild hay fever, perennial

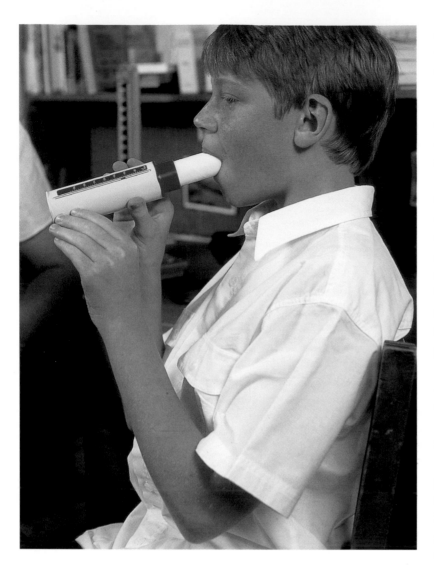

Monitoring the airways of an asthma sufferer using a peak-flow meter is important both for the diagnosis and management of the condition.

rhinitis, and conjunctivitis, and it is the main treatment for urticaria and simple angioedema (see p. 20).

Antihistamines, as their name suggests, oppose the effects of histamine within the body. Histamine is one of the major chemicals released as part of an allergic reaction and it is an important contributor to the development of symptoms.

There are several ways that histamine can act, and in allergy it is the H1-antihistamines that are used as a treatment. This treatment reduces the itching, the generation of secretions (watery eyes or runny nose), and also sneezing, but it has less effect on obstructive symptoms, such as a blocked nose. Asthmatic conditions, too, are less responsive. In general H1-antihistamines are not used for asthma.

A range of different antihistamines is available, some with sedative effects and some without. Since sedative antihistamines can have the side-effect of impairing your social interactions, driving skills, and your ability to concentrate at school or at work, the non-sedating antihistamines should be used in tablet form to relieve symptoms during daytime activities.

Antileukotrienes Another class of drugs that can be used to fight the symptoms of allergy is antileukotrines. Leukotrienes are important chemicals released by the body during an allergic episode and other inflammatory reactions. The introduction of antileukotrines widens the airways and improves symptoms in asthma. These drugs may also modify some aspects of the underlying inflammation in the airway, but this is still being evaluated. As leukotrines are only part of the allergic reaction, treatment combining both antileukotrines and other drugs, such as H1-antihistamines, is being researched to see if this provides greater benefit.

Anti-inflammatory therapy The development of allergic inflammation is the underlying basis for asthma, rhinitis, conjunctivitis, and eczema. Drugs that suppress this inflammation provide the most effective method of relieving symptoms. The main anti-inflammatory drugs are the corticosteroids, although chromones are also used. Corticosteroids are administered via the nose, airways, eyes, or skin in the form of a spray, as an inhaled aerosol, drops, or as a cream or ointment for the treatment of rhinitis, asthma, conjunctivitis, and eczema, respectively. Steroids can also be given orally for these conditions, as well as for urticaria, depending on the severity. External/inhaled application is preferable since lower doses are then required and there is less concern about any potential side-effects with long-term use.

This treatment needs to be taken on a daily basis to suppress the inflammation and is considered to be a preventer, or prophylactic, therapy. Other forms of treatment are needed for the acute relief of symptoms.

Reliever therapy In general, the term reliever therapy is used to describe medication taken by asthma sufferers when needed to relax the muscles around their airways that have been constricted due to the inflammation, and so make their breathing easier. Drugs that fall into this category are usually given by inhalation (*see below right*), rather than orally, for rapid effect. Short-acting types are used as a medication whenever someone with asthma feels uncomfortable with their breathing. The long-acting varieties, which last 12 hours, are used regularly, twice daily or at bedtime to prevent the airways narrowing and so minimize symptoms. These drugs should be used in conjunction with an anti-inflammatory.

Theophylline therapy is also designed to widen the airways and ease breathing. The medication is taken, by mouth, on a daily basis as a maintenance treatment to minimize symptoms. Theophyllines are generally used as an add-on therapy to preventer therapies for people suffering with asthma. They have a very narrow therapeutic to toxicity ratio and must not be taken without a physician's recommendation.

Immunotherapy

Immnotherapy involves being given repeated injections of increasingly larger doses of an allergen to which you are sensitized. The aim is to alter your immune system's response to that specific allergen and decrease its response to the offending allergen(s). Such treatment requires a long term commitment: injections are weekly or biweekly to start with, and the treatment can last between three and five years. Since serious reactions can arise in response to these injections, they should be undertaken by an allergy specialist.

If successful, this treatment is, however, the only one (apart from allergen avoidance) that can fundamentally alter the allergic response. It has been shown to be most effective for pollen-allergy sufferers, but has limited and variable success with combating other forms of allergy.

Your suitability for immunotherapy treatment would have to be assessed by a specialist.

Alternative approaches to injected allergens are being assessed.

Management of anaphylaxis

Anaphylaxis is such an extreme medical condition that the identification of the offending agent and then the strictest possible regime of avoidance is the only effective basis of treatment. This is such an acute condition that if, for any reason, total avoidance is not possible or an accidental exposure occurs, all anaphylaxis sufferers should be provided with, and be instructed on how to use, a pre-loaded adrenaline syringe for self-administration.

Adrenaline is the most important drug for the management of anaphylaxis. Patients should carry this with them all the time. The early use of adrenaline can be life-saving.

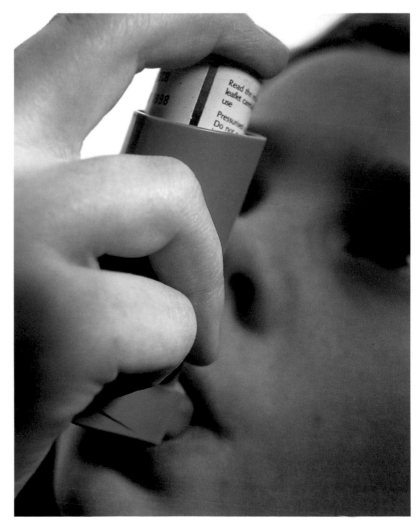

Inhalers, which are available in many different designs, are a standard method of administering drugs to the airways both to prevent and relieve the symptoms of asthma.

The Allergy-Free Home

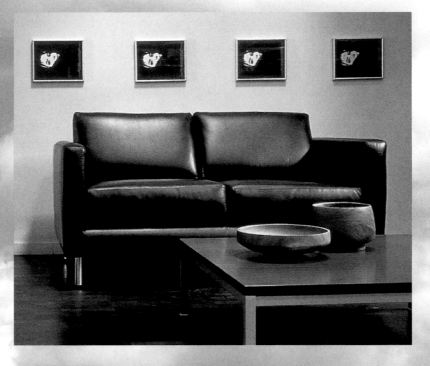

Indoor Air Quality

The interior environment is the main place where people are exposed to the allergens that result in such common allergic conditions as asthma, rhinitis, and eczema. Many of these allergens, including animal dander and mould spores, are found in the air, while others, such as mite droppings, are in carpets and bedding, but become airborne if disturbed.

In addition, the air in buildings contains other pollutants, such as the sulphur dioxide given off by burning fuel, that do not cause allergies in themselves but may make the symptoms of allergic diseases worse.

Research has shown that air inside is often more polluted than that outside. Indeed, the levels of some pollutants can be as much as 20–30 times higher indoors. These findings are even more important when you realize that most people spend between 75 and 90 percent of their time indoors.

Studies of air pollution in buildings have found the following:

- House-dust mite allergen
- Cockroach allergen
- Mould spores
- Pet dander
- Pollen
- Combustion by-products, such as carbon monoxide, nitrogen oxides, and sulphur dioxide
- Tobacco smoke
- Chemicals given off by home improvement and household products
- Bacteria and viruses
- Trace metals
- Pesticides

Pollutants – allergen or irritant?

Some interior air pollutants, such as cat dander, are allergens and it is these that cause allergic symptoms. Cat dander can be very persistent and may still be found in a home several years after a cat has lived there. Other inside pollutants, such as solvents from paints, are irritants, and these may provoke or worsen allergic symptoms in some individuals who already have a lowered tolerance threshold for airborne substances as a result of their allergic condition.

High humidity is another factor affecting air quality. We all feel lethargic and uncomfortable when humidity levels are high. But more than this, if high humidity is allowed to persist for long periods, it will cause damp and rot that may affect your furniture and fittings. High humidity will also encourage the growth of mould and the spread of dust mites.

Causes of interior air pollution

Air pollution in buildings is partly the result of poor ventilation (see pp. 52–3), which allows air pollutants to build up to high levels. Over the years, homes have become increasingly energy efficient through the addition of double- (secondary-) glazing, draught-proofing (weather stripping), and insulation. Central heating has also replaced open fires, with the result that most chimneys have been either removed or blocked up. Although homes are now warmer, open fires used to create a draught of

fresh air through the house and up the chimneys, so that stale interior air was continually refreshed with outdoor air.

Many chemicals are found in the modern home as part of cleaning, hobby, or home improvement products, or have been included in the manufacturing process of carpets, clothes, and furniture. And many of these are released in small amounts into the air (out-gassed), sometimes for months or years, producing a spectrum of interior air pollutants for us all to contend with. For example, homes built in the 1980s are more likely to have higher levels of the gas formaldehyde (see pp. 68–9) than older homes, which are less likely to have modern, board-based furniture (see pp. 70–1). Another important group of interior air pollutants are volatile organic compounds (VOCs), which are given off by many household and cleaning products (see pp. 68–9).

Improving interior air quality

Ventilation is the key to improving the quality of the air we breathe inside. This may mean opening windows or installing an extractor (exhaust) fan in the kitchen and bathroom, or upgrading the filter in our air-conditioning. More comprehensive action may include installing a full or half-house ventilation system (see pp. 56–7). Even the choices we make when decorating and cleaning our homes (see pp. 62–7) have an effect on air quality.

Better air quality, which can in many cases be provided naturally simply by opening doors or windows, benefits everybody, not just those with allergies or other breathing difficulties.

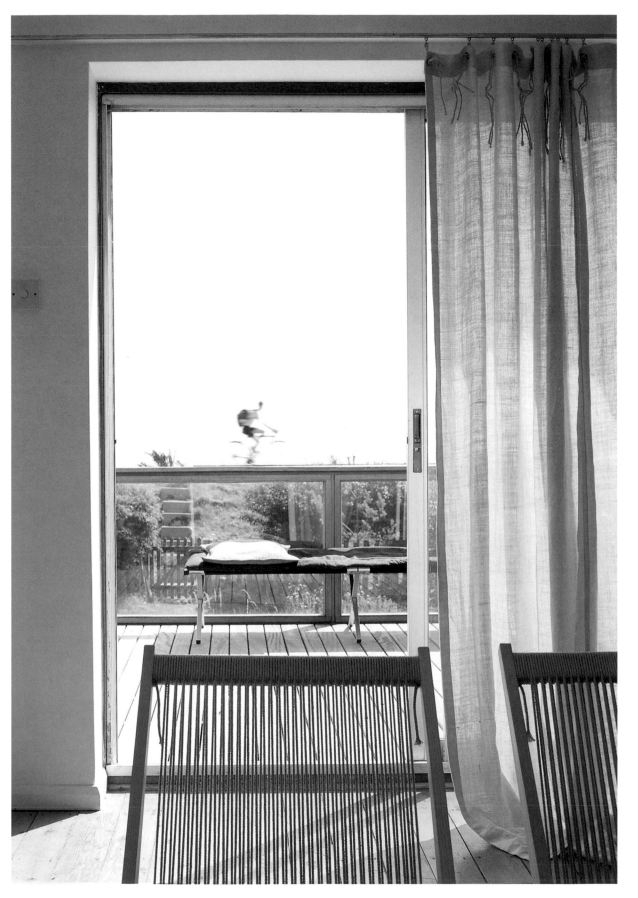

VENTILATION AND HUMIDITY

Good ventilation involves removing stale, polluted air from a house and replacing it with less-polluted air from outside. One of the main functions of ventilation is removing excess humidity (water vapour in the air), with the average family producing a surprisingly large amount (*see below*). Other functions of ventilation include removing interior air pollutants, such as those produced during cooking, replacing oxygen as it is breathed in and used up, and removing carbon dioxide as it is breathed out.

Problems due to poor ventilation can occur when people try to "do the right thing" by introducing such energy-conservation measures as insulation and double- (secondary-) glazing. These measures seal up some of the normal routes of air into and out of the home, so reducing ventilation. As a result, this may lead to high levels of humidity and air pollutants.

Moisture sources in a 4-person household

Source	Moisture produced (litres/pints)
Four people asleep for 8 hours	1–2/1¾–3½
Two people active for 16 hours	1.5–3/2½–5¼
Cooking per 24 hours	2–4/3½–7
Bathing and dish washing per 24 hours	0.5–1/¾–1¾
Washing clothes per 24 hours	0.5–1/¾–1¾
Use of unvented tumble dryers per 24 hours	3–7.5/2½–13¼
Paraffin heater per 24 hours	1–2/1¾–3½

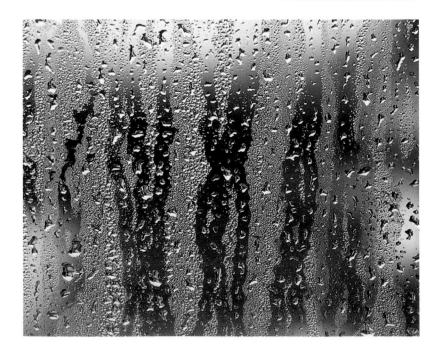

What is humidity?

Air always contains some water in the form of an invisible vapour. The amount of water that air can hold increases with temperature, so that hot air can potentially hold more water vapour than cold. However, whatever the air temperature, there comes a point at which the air can absorb no more water vapour and it is then said to be saturated.

Relative humidity gives us an idea of how saturated the air is at a particular temperature and so how much more water vapour it can still absorb. Air with a relative humidity of 100 percent is completely saturated and can absorb no more vapour, while air with a relative humidity of 50 percent can absorb twice as much before reaching saturation.

Air with a low relative humidity feels dry and can absorb much more water vapour than air with a higher relative humidity. Dry air is bad news for the house-dust mite, as a low relative humidity makes it harder for the mite to absorb the moisture it needs from the air. Thus, mites grow better at a high relative humidity, as do moulds. Moisture is more likely to condense at a high relative humidity on to cold surfaces, such as windowsills, where mould will grow if the water is not wiped away. Persistently high relative humidity also encourages the emission (out-gassing) of chemicals from products in the home.

High relative humidity is perceived as being uncomfortably muggy. The comfort zone for people is between

Wipe away condensation to prevent mould growth and rot, or open the window until the condensation has cleared.

Common causes of damp

Rising damp	Water rises up from the ground because of a faulty or missing damp-proof course. In some situations, even though the damp-proof course is intact, it may have been bridged by plaster or rendering (stucco) on the outside of the building.
Penetrating damp	Water comes through the wall after heavy rain. This is often caused by a leaking gutter or downpipe (downspout). If the damp is low down, soil may have been heaped against the wall above the damp-proof course. Penetrating damp is more likely to affect old, solid walls rather than modern, cavity walls.
Condensation	Water condenses from humid air and settles on cold surfaces or in cold corners in poorly heated and badly ventilated rooms.

40 and 70 percent relative humidity, while the breeding rate of house-dust mites is reduced once relative humidity falls below 70 percent.

Taking basic action

By taking the following into account any remedial action you take to improve ventilation will be more effective.

Defeating damp Identify and deal with sources of damp. The main causes are penetrating damp, rising damp, and condensation (see above). It is not always easy to diagnose what may be the cause(s), and even specialists don't always get it right, so obtain professional advice from several specialist companies.

Improving insulation Adding basic insulation will make your home warmer, more comfortable, and less expensive to run. Insulation will also help to eliminate, or minimize, cold spots, which, in turn, will reduce condensation and associated mould growth.

Draught-proofing (or weather stripping) If you make your home more airtight you will increase its comfort and save on energy. Draught-proofing (weather stripping) doors and

windows is a good start, but there are other ways by which you can influence the amount of air that passes in and out of your home:

- When decorating, seal gaps under skirting (base) boards, around the edge of window frames, and under windowsills
- Check the ceiling for gaps where pipes enter the attic (loft) and draught-proof (weather strip) around the attic (loft) entrance
- Fill the cavity of the outside walls with insulation to stop unwanted air leakage, as well as reducing heat loss

However, having done this, you will then need to pay more attention to your home's ventilation to make sure that you have the right amount of air in the right place and at the right time.

Creating natural ventilation

All homes have some degree of natural ventilation. The wind blows through spaces in the building's structure – through the walls and gaps in windows, under doors, and so on. In addition, the natural rising of warm air and its exit from the top of a building pulls in fresh air from outside – an effect known as stack ventilation.

In temperate climates (warm, wet winters and hot, drier summers), natural ventilation may often be enough to reduce humidity and dilute indoor pollutants to tolerable levels. You should, therefore, try sleeping with your bedroom windows slightly open, or at least open them when you first get up. This will reduce humidity, especially in winter, by bringing fresh, colder air in, and so help to reduce the mite population, which needs high humidity to thrive.

However, leaving windows open at night may not be advisable if cold weather induces asthma symptoms. In this case, air the bedroom well at other times of the day. If you suffer from a pollen allergy (see pp. 28–31), also keep windows shut at night during the pollen season. Air the room during the afternoon, when the pollen count is usually at its lowest.

In addition, you should always open windows in the bathroom after bathing and in the kitchen when you are cooking to allow the moisture-laden air to escape to the outside. However, keep the doors to these rooms shut during use to prevent moisture from escaping into the rest of the home.

IMPROVING VENTILATION

Natural ventilation has its shortcoming: on days when there is little wind, some parts of the house will be poorly ventilated; on cold days, the incoming air may be too cold for comfort; or you may have hay fever and need to shut windows during the pollen season. The effects of inadequate ventilation include increased interior humidity and higher levels of interior pollutants (*see pp. 50–3*).

However, you can take steps to improve ventilation. These include fitting air vents in windows to increase background ventilation, and extractor (exhaust) fans in the kitchen and bathroom to remove moisture. Alternatively, you may want to install a mechanical ventilation system (*see pp. 56–7*).

Can a mechanical ventilation system help me?

The answer to this question is probably "yes". The range of benefits an efficient, well-installed mechanical ventilation system can bring include: a continual renewal of stale inside air with fresher air from outside; reduced levels of pollutants in the home; and the option to close up your home during times of peak pollen counts or high pollution levels. Depending on the allergens and irritants that trigger your allergic symptoms, such a system may be worth considering for these reasons alone.

To see how a mechanical ventilation system could reduce the severity or frequency of allergic symptoms, you have to look more closely at what a system could do. A reasonable expectation is that it actively refreshes the air right through your home by extracting stale air inside and replacing it with fresher air from outside. In addition, during winter, a ventilation system is likely to help decrease house-dust mite numbers by bringing in cold air from outside, so lowering relative humidity inside.

Research suggests that in countries with several months of very cold weather, mechanical ventilation alone can greatly reduce house-dust mite numbers. An explanation could be that the long period of low relative humidity during the winter so reduces the mite population that it cannot recover during the warmer, more humid summer months.

In more temperate climates, recent studies have shown that despite shorter, warmer winters, a mechanical ventilation system will reduce mite-allergen levels in the home.

If you are sensitive to mites, you need to bear in mind that a mechanical ventilation system can help only if it is part of an overall dust-mite management programme, including such elements as anti-mite barrier covers on bedding (*see pp. 88–9*) and mite-unfriendly furnishings and floor surfaces (*see pp. 70–1 and 63–4*).

Ventilation requirements

When looking at ventilation for your own home, any action you take should be guided by modern building regulations, which are designed to make sure there is sufficient ventilation to reduce potential damage due to condensation and to promote better interior air quality.

Following the guidelines given in the box (*see right*), the action in step 1 should be enough for most homes. You may want to add a single-room

BETTER VENTILATION

Following the advice in Step 1 should be satisfactory for most homes, but see Step 2 if you have an allergy sufferer in your home. Step 3 provides an excellent level of ventilation, but the cost involved needs to be considered critically against any extra health benefits.

Step 1
- Install extractor (exhaust) fans in the kitchen and bathroom and fit air grilles (trickle ventilators) into the window frames of bedrooms and living rooms, or fit security locks that allow windows to be left safely ajar.
- Leave bedroom trickle ventilators open in all but the coldest, windiest weather to ensure a supply of outside air to help keep humidity low.
- Fit an overrun timer to the bathroom extractor (exhaust) fan and use it every time you have a bath or shower. Turn the fan on before the tap (faucet).

Step 2
- Add a single-room ventilation unit to critical rooms, for example the bedroom of an asthmatic.

Step 3
- Consider mechanical ventilation with heat recovery.
- If this is not possible, install a partial-house system serving upstairs only (*see p. 57*).

ventilation unit to the bedroom of someone with an allergy (step 2), while step 3 is usually only carried out when remodelling your house.

Each room of your home should have some form of "rapid" and "background" natural ventilation. Rapid

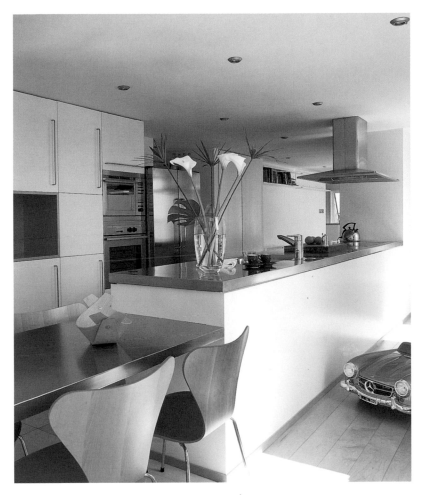

ventilation can be provided in the form of an opening window. This is not difficult in most rooms, but some toilets and bathrooms may have fixed windows or none at all. In this case, you will need to fit an extractor (exhaust) fan (see *below*).

Background ventilation is provided by a small opening that can be left open – one that does not let in rain or burglars. In homes with modern windows, this will usually be a trickle ventilator – a small air grille set into the window frame. In other homes, you may need to install trickle ventilators or put in security locks that allow windows to be left safely ajar.

"Extract" ventilation   In "wet" rooms – those rooms that produce a lot of moisture, such as kitchens, bathrooms, and laundry rooms – you should have a method of extracting water-laden air, probably via an extractor (exhaust) fan, although passive ventilation systems are used in some countries (see *p. 57*).

Extractor (exhaust) fans or hoods

The quietness and efficiency of modern extractor (exhaust) fans or hoods make them an attractive proposition. They must, however, discharge air to the outside rather than into any internal space or attached garage, otherwise problems of condensation and even mould and rot may occur.

The fan is best positioned on an outside wall, away from the room door or window, which should be closed when the fan is on, otherwise air will come in through the window or door and go straight out again via the fan, leaving the room essentially unventilated. Some fans have an automatic control that switches them

to high speed when the room humidity rises above a preset level. At low humidities, the fan turns off, or operates at low speed. Low-voltage splash-proof fans are available for wet areas, such as inside a shower cubicle. Extractor (exhaust) fans may also be installed in garages, home offices, and workshops to remove fumes.

Boilers or heating appliances

An open-flued appliance draws the air it needs from inside the home. A lack of air will cause inadequate combustion, an increase in the amount of carbon monoxide, and a greater risk of combustion by-products leaking into the room.

These by-products provoke such symptoms as sneezing or coughing

There should be some way of extracting air from rooms that produce a lot of moisture, such as the kitchen, often done by installing a hood over the cooker (stove). The hood should be vented to the outside (see p. 97).

in some people with respiratory allergies, but there is also the danger of carbon monoxide poisoning. Both these potential problems are avoided with balanced-flue appliances, which draw their air directly from outside and exhaust all their combustion by-products outside (see *pp. 60–1*).

There should not be an extractor (exhaust) fan or vented cooker (stove) hood in the same room as an open-flued appliance, as the draught of air going out through the extractor may suck air, along with any combustion by-products, back down the flue of the appliance and into the room.

VENTILATION SYSTEMS

The most comprehensive form of mechanical ventilation is "mechanical ventilation with heat recovery", or MVHR (*see below*). It is easily installed in houses under construction or in existing, single-storey homes. Existing, multi-storey homes may benefit from a partial-house system (see *opposite*).

For maximum benefit, your home must be well insulated and reasonably airtight. There is little point in paying for a sophisticated system if your house is full of draughts. The company fitting the system should include draught-proofing (weather stripping) as part of the installation procedure.

How MVHR works

The system comprises a central unit containing an exhaust fan, inlet fan, and a heat-exchanger. It supplies fresh air via ducting and air inlets to all living rooms and bedrooms, while extracting stale air from the kitchen and bathroom and exhausting it to the

Installing an MVHR system

Siting the heat-recovery unit	● Choose a position, commonly in the attic (loft), near the middle of the house. This usually provides the shortest route (and least expense) for ducting. ● Make sure that the chosen location allows access for servicing the heat-recovery unit. Fans, filters, and the heat-exchanger need regular cleaning to maintain their operation at peak efficiency. ● Consider designs that locate the heat-recovery unit over the cooker (stove) and incorporate a hood. This makes the fan and filters easily accessible. ● Don't site the inlet or outlet on a wall facing the prevailing wind if your home is on a windy site. ● Keep inlets and outlets well apart to avoid cross-contamination of airflows.
Installing ducting	● Avoid sharp bends in the ducting to prevent reducing efficiency. ● Hide ducting inside built-in cabinets or in a boxed-in corner. ● If the unit is in the attic (loft), insulate the ducts between the unit and the point where they enter the warm house. If the unit is inside the house, insulate the ducts between the unit and the outside.
Siting supply inlets and extract outlets	● Site a supply inlet in every "dry" room to ensure correct total airflow distribution. ● Avoid inlets or outlets in hallways or landings, as this may interfere with the airflow. ● Locate supply inlets opposite doors to ensure airflow throughout the whole room. ● If your house has large rooms, it is best to install one supply inlet at each end of the room.
Catering for adequate air exchange	● The required air-exchange rate depends on the number of people and lifestyle. ● For best results, your house should be as airtight as possible. ● Leave gaps at the bottom of internal doors to allow air to circulate. ● Consider running the ventilation system continuously – especially at night, which is one of the worst times for condensation. ● If in doubt about any aspect, speak to a specialist installer or advisory body.
Maintenance	● Maintain ventilation systems scrupulously to avoid the recirculation of pollutants and microorganisms from clogged filters or ducts.

Characteristics of air filters

Activated charcoal	Specially treated, very porous charcoal. A gaseous filter that removes most volatile organic compounds, but not formaldehyde, and therefore activated alumina, which can absorb formaldehyde, is sometimes added.
Extended surface	A particulate filter made from fibreglass or polyester fibres held together by a synthetic resin. Filters out many airborne particles and pollens.
HEPA (high-efficiency particulate air)	A very powerful extended-surface particulate filter capable of removing 97 percent or more of particles as small as 0.3 microns. These filters are necessary if you wish to eliminate smoke from the air. Since smoke contains both particulates and gases, an activated charcoal filter will also be needed.
Electrostatic	A plastic, particulate filter that relies on static electricity to capture particulates. Some can be cleaned and reused but others must be replaced when dirty. Fairly efficient at removing larger particles such as pollen and mould spores, but not efficient at removing particles smaller than 6 microns.
Electrostatic precipitator	Strictly speaking, this is not a filter at all, since the air does not pass through any type of filtering material. It is connected to the home's electrical system and imparts a negative charge to particles, such as dust, mould spores, and pollen grains in the airstream, so that they become attracted to a positively charged collecting plate. The plate has to be regularly washed to maintain its operating efficiency.

outside. The unit contains a heat-exchanger, which ensures that the warm, stale air gives up most of its heat to the incoming air. The air brought in from outside is filtered before being dispersed around the home.

Thus, the living and bedrooms receive a continuous supply of prewarmed, filtered, fresh air, while moisture and odours are removed from the kitchen and bathroom.

Choice of filters An air filter cleans the air by physically removing substances from it as it passes through the filter. Filters are either particulate, removing particles such as mould, pollen, dust, bacteria, and viruses, or gaseous, removing gases and vapours such as carbon monoxide and formaldehyde. They also vary in the range of particles or gases filtered,

with more efficient filters being better for low-allergen homes. Air filters are also used in forced-air heating and air-conditioning systems, air-filtering units (see pp. 58–9), and vacuum cleaners (see pp. 74–5). Clean and change filters as recommended to avoid contamination with bacteria and mould.

Partial-house systems

In an existing, multi-storey home a partial ventilation system may help to improve interior air quality, provided the building has been effectively draught-proofed. A partial system supplies air to upstairs bedrooms and extracts air from the bathroom. Stale, polluted air, working its way up from below, is extracted from the landing area. The system is supplemented by a kitchen range or cooker (stove) hood downstairs, and also by a single-room

heat-recovery ventilation unit or air inlets in the living rooms.

Single-room units

This ventilation system combines a supply fan, exhaust fan, and heat-exchanger in an easily installed unit. It may help to control humidity and air quality in a single room, such as the bedroom of an allergy sufferer.

Passive stack ventilation

In this system, warm, moist air rises up through ducts leading from the kitchen and bathroom ceilings to outlets in the roof. Fresh air entering through grilles in the living room and bedrooms replaces this stale, moisture-laden air. Stack ventilation uses no fans and depends solely on the fact that warm air rises. It is best installed in new homes when they are being built.

PORTABLE AIR-QUALITY UNITS

Air-filtering units and ionizers are sometimes promoted as being helpful to people with allergies. While research shows that air-filtering units fitted with HEPA filters (see p. 57) may help asthma symptoms if they are used with anti-mite bedding covers (see pp. 88–9), there is no evidence that ionizers reduce allergic symptoms. Dehumidifiers and air-conditioning units may be helpful in certain situations, but humidifiers are likely to cause problems for those with allergies.

Air-filtering units

These units work by trapping pollutants as air is drawn by a fan through special filters (see p. 57). These units were originally designed for removing pollutants, such as tobacco smoke, from small, localized areas – such as you might find in an office reception area, where the general background noise would mask the sound of the filtering unit.

There is some doubt concerning the effectiveness of these units in removing mite allergen, but this is probably because of the type of filters used. Research shows that if fitted with HEPA filters they do improve the symptoms of mite-sensitive asthma when used together with anti-mite bedding. However, it is vital to concentrate on controlling mites by removing carpets and improving ventilation, and on measures that make sure that there is less dust in the air (see pp. 72–5).

If you are interested in an air-filtering unit, opt for the model with the most powerful fan and an HEPA filter. Other factors to consider when buying a unit include how noisy it is when operating and how often you have to change filters.

Dehumidifiers

The way dehumidifiers work is by cooling air so that excess humidity condenses into a container, to be emptied either automatically or manually. Whole-house dehumidifiers are available that claim to reduce relative humidity in the home to below 50 percent. If true, they are likely to have an effect on mould growth and mite numbers. In summer, however, the heat given out by a dehumidifier can make the house too warm, so that air conditioning is also needed.

Smaller units may be helpful in drying out a flooded or newly plastered room, but are unlikely to play a major role in improving air quality.

Humidifiers

These units add moisture to the air. Since normal human activity produces a lot of water vapour (see p. 52), it is usually unwise to put extra humidity into the air. From a health point of view, too dry is usually better than too humid. People sometimes complain that the air dries out when the central heating is on. However, this is because the relative humidity has been lowered (see p. 52) and not because the central heating has removed moisture from the air. Using a humidifier may make the air feel more comfortable,

---

MAKING THE MOST OF IONIZERS

Although some people report an improvement in symptoms with an ionizer in use, many years of research have failed to provide any clear scientific evidence that they help. Older models made asthma symptoms worse in some people because the small amount of ozone they produced irritated the airways, but this problem has been rectified in new models.

Ionizers are effective at removing particles, such as mould spores, from the air, although their range is limited. The particles removed settle on surfaces, such as walls or furniture, from where they can be hard to remove. Some people hang a curtain behind the

ionizer to help catch the dirt removed by the ionizer unit.

If you do decide to try an ionizer, following these tips should help the ionizer to clean the air better:
- Place the ionizer at the very front edge of an easy-to-clean, non-metal surface, well off the ground and away from the walls.
- Point the ionizer into the room and keep objects away from its front or sides.
- Never clean it with furniture polish as this may interfere with the way it works. Use a damp (not wet) cloth instead.

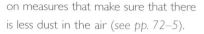

Once combined with the ions emitted by an ionizer, airborne mould spores, pollen, and dust become attracted to surfaces, such as walls or ceilings, leaving the air cleaner.

THE HOUSE PLANT CONTROVERSY

There has been much speculation about the ability of house plants to act as air filters. Studies in the 1980s, sponsored by NASA as part of their space research programme, suggested some house plants were effective at removing volatile organic compounds, including formaldehyde, from air in buildings. The studies were carried out in sealed test chambers and later in a small, tightly sealed structure called the "Biohome".

Some researchers have failed to replicate these results, while others have claimed to have reproduced them. In recent years, several high-profile plant-based air and waste-water purification systems have been designed and installed in public buildings. However, the use of plants as part of an ecologically designed system to create a healthy indoor environment is still in its infancy. Further evidence is needed on just how plants might be used to improve the home environment. Meanwhile, it should be kept in mind that, whatever their air-cleaning ability, plants increase humidity and moulds may grow in the soil.

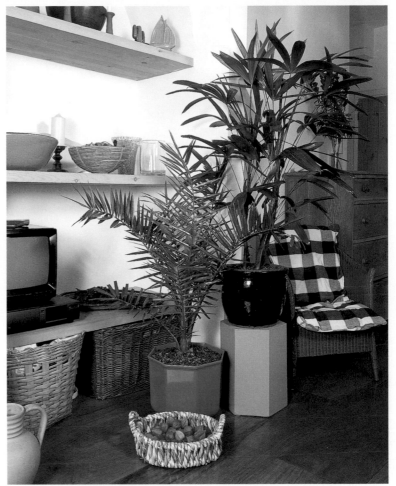

but you will be providing more favourable conditions for mould and dust mites. Try setting your central heating to a lower temperature instead.

In addition, humidifiers contain a reservoir of standing water, which can become the breeding ground for bacteria and mould. Even if the unit has been designed to kill these microorganisms, dead allergenic mould may still be blown out along with the humidified air.

Humidifiers can be used to help medical conditions, such as croup, but steam inhalation is as effective. If a child with asthma is having breathing problems at night, the cause should be sought and dealt with by your doctor.

Air-conditioning units

Most domestic air-conditioning systems, including stand-alone units, simply cool and recirculate the air within the area they operate; they do not necessarily bring fresh air in from outside. This is not always realized – because stand-alone air conditioners are often mounted through a window, people assume that they exchange interior with exterior air as part of their operation. In fact, window mounting is simply the easiest method of exhausting the heat they take from inside the home.

Stand-alone units do not usually have any air filters, while filters provided for central air-conditioning

systems are primarily designed to protect the cooling unit, and need upgrading if they are to be of any benefit to allergy sufferers.

Regular maintenance of stand-alone units (and the ductwork of central systems) prevents a build-up of dust and contamination by mould and bacteria – running the unit for 30 minutes after turning off the cooling function helps to dry out the system and prevent mould growth.

Air conditioning may benefit pollen sufferers, as windows can be kept closed during peak pollen times. Air conditioning also helps to reduce relative humidity, so helping to control dust mite numbers and mould growth.

Heating

Only a generation ago we would have kept warm by the kitchen range or an open fire in the living room, while the rest of the home would have been much cooler. Today, modern heating systems allow us to walk around any room during winter wearing comfortable, lightweight clothing.

There is, however, more than a monetary price to pay for the benefits we derive from our heating systems – the environment they create is ideal for the house-dust mite (*see pp. 36–7*). Warmer houses, together with increased humidity, carpeting, and soft furnishings, have encouraged the mite population to expand – particularly in bedrooms, where we spend about a third of our lives.

At the same time, draught-proofing (weather stripping) and insulation – to keep in all that extra heat – have dramatically decreased ventilation (*see pp. 52–7*), resulting in higher levels of interior pollutants. These include those produced by burning fuel, which are

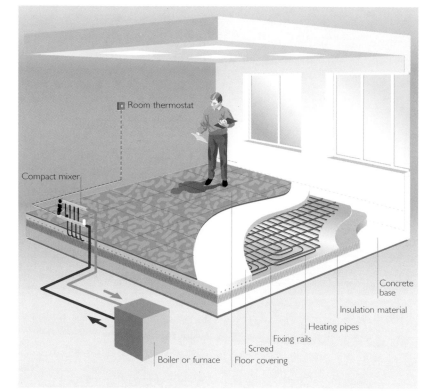

Room thermostat
Compact mixer
Concrete base
Insulation material
Heating pipes
Fixing rails
Screed
Boiler or furnace
Floor covering

often described as combustion by-products (*see below*). High levels of these gases, such as sulphur dioxide, can make asthmatic conditions worse.

In underfloor heating, insulating material is laid underneath the pipes, which are covered with a lightweight screed. Hot water from a boiler or furnace, at the temperature set on the room thermostat, is fed to the pipes,

COMBUSTION SOURCES AND COMBUSTION BY-PRODUCTS

Each combustion source produces by-products. Reducing the overall number of sources in the home lowers levels of combustion gases.

COMMON SOURCES
- Coal-burning fires
- Wood stoves or open fires
- Gas cookers (stoves) or ranges
- Gas clothes dryers
- Gas- and oil-fuelled water heaters, furnaces, or boilers
- Butane or propane gas heaters
- Kerosene (paraffin) heaters
- Oil lamps

- Candles and aromatherapy lamps
- Tobacco smoking

COMBUSTION BY-PRODUCTS
- Water
- Nitrogen dioxide
- Nitrogen oxides
- Sulphur dioxide
- Hydrogen cyanide
- Carbon monoxide
- Carbon dioxide
- Formaldehyde
- Hydrocarbons, such as butane, propane, benzene
- Particulate matter

Combustion appliances

As a result of the combustion of fuel, certain by-products are inevitably produced, including water, solid particles (particulates), and, depending on the fuel being burned, a range of gases (*see left*). This occurs with all appliances that burn fuel. If these by-products are released into the air in the building, they may provoke respiratory symptoms, such as sneezing, coughing, or even an asthma attack, in some people with rhinitis or asthma. High levels of nitrogen oxides may also increase the number of respiratory infections in children. The following points will help you to minimize the level of combustion by-products in the home:

● Keep the number of combustion appliances in the home to a minimum
● Have combustion appliances serviced regularly – once a year
● Make sure that chimneys and flues are working properly
● Keep your home well ventilated

Boilers or furnaces Balanced-flue boilers, or furnaces, are sealed off from the room. They draw the air they need to burn their fuel from outside, which is where they also exhaust all their combustion by-products. This system is the preferred type for a low-allergen home.

Other boilers or furnaces are open-flued (see p. 55). With these systems, the flue is open to the room from which it draws its air. This means that the combustion gases may escape back into the room.

Unflued heaters Portable liquid-propane gas, paraffin (kerosene), or butane gas heaters have no place in the low-allergen home. They are unflued and so emit combustion by-products straight into the interior air. In addition, they increase humidity due to the amount of water they produce as a result of combustion. Similarly, unflued gas convector heaters should not be fitted in the low-allergen home.

Heating methods

Although there are many types of heat-delivery system for the home, they are all either mainly convection or radiant in the way they do their job.

Convection heating systems circulate heated air around a room,

---

MINIMIZING COMBUSTION BY-PRODUCTS

● Stop smoking. Passive smoking by children increases the respiratory infections they contract and worsens the symptoms of asthma. If you find it impossible to quit, set aside a well-ventilated "smoking room", perhaps fitted with an air filter unit or an extractor fan.
● Consider replacing open fires with imitation coal or wood electric fires. Avoid gas fires.
● Make sure that chimneys are functioning properly – it is important that there is an adequate supply of replacement air available for that used up during combustion.
● When the time comes to replace your gas cooker (stove), consider buying an electric model.
● If you must cook with gas, make sure that your hood is sufficiently powerful to remove by-products

and that it is installed at the correct height for best effect.
● Consider installing a high-efficiency gas or oil boiler or furnace with a sealed combustion chamber, which blows by-products outside through a sealed exhaust pipe.
● Have boilers and fuel-burning appliances serviced once a year.
● Do not use bottled gas heaters (butane and propane) or paraffin (kerosene) heaters, since these produce a lot of water vapour during combustion, as well as combustion products that are emitted into the interior air.
● Vent gas-fuelled clothes dryers to the outside, or dry clothes outside when possible.
● Use incense burners, candles, or aromatherapy oils only in a properly ventilated room (see pp. 52–7).

---

taking with it allergen-containing dust particles. Radiant heating, however, warms the air directly and so does not disturb the dust. Radiant heating is also preferred because it prevents "cold spots", thus reducing mould growth and dust-mite numbers.

Forced-air heating systems These systems have a poor reputation for blowing dust around. However, if you regularly vacuum (see pp. 74–5), there should be less dust to become a problem. Remember to maintain and clear a forced-air system regularly, especially the ducting, to prevent the build up of dust, mould, and bacteria.

Conventional radiators As long as you vacuum regularly underneath and behind the units to prevent dust building up, conventional radiators, which heat mainly by convection, can be satisfactory in a low-allergen home.

Underfloor heating In underfloor heating, heated water is passed through pipes laid under the floor (see left). The heat is mainly radiant, so that the air and, therefore, dust is left un-disturbed. Underfloor heating makes hard-surface floors, such as wood, more comfortable, and may possibly keep carpets too dry for house-dust mites (and mould). It is best installed when a house is being built, or when a floor is being laid as part of rebuilding, such as a house-extension project.

Radiant skirting (base) boards This method of radiant heating can be installed in existing homes. The normal, solid skirting (base) board is replaced with a hollow one containing either heated-water pipes connected to a boiler or electrically heated pipes. The heated skirting (base) board radiates heat evenly through the room and does not disturb dust.

Floors and Walls

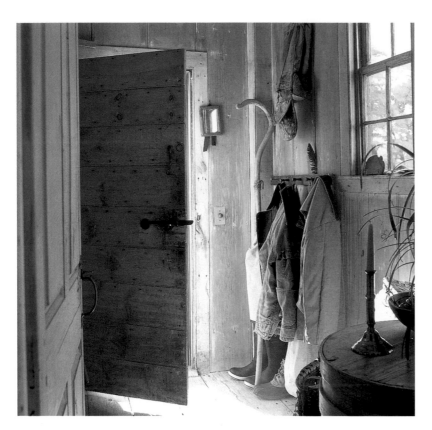

Mould spores and pollen, as well as other contaminants, are easily brought inside on your shoes. Adopt a "no-shoes" policy inside the house to keep dirt and outdoor allergens outside.

Microscopically small allergen particles in the home will settle on all fabrics and surfaces – not just on horizontal surfaces, such as floors, ledges, and shelves, but also vertical ones, such as walls. Depending on the type of covering, floors in particular are potentially a major allergen reservoir. If you are serious about maintaining a low-allergen home, this can be difficult to achieve with carpets. They are not easy to clean thoroughly and they provide the ideal habitat for house-dust mites (see pp. 36–7), as well as collecting dirt and other allergens, such as mould spores and pollen.

Fitted carpets

Wall-to-wall carpeting is today's most popular flooring material, and can also be the unhealthiest. A look through a microscope reveals microorganisms covering every strand and fibre. Although many of these organisms represent no danger to human health,

there are some – particularly house-dust mites and mould spores – that are major causes of allergies.

Soon after a new carpet has been installed, house-dust mites will be busy making themselves at home. Micro-organisms, such as bacteria and moulds, can also thrive in carpeting, which provides them with a warm, moist environment with plenty to eat. Dirt will inevitably be walked into the carpet from outside, depositing traces of soil, pollen, animal dander, animal waste products, pesticide residues, mould spores, and so on. This is a good reason to adopt a "no-shoes" policy in the home, for guests as well as members of the family.

Children are most at risk from soiled carpeting. Adults usually sit on chairs or sofas and are unlikely to come into direct contact with the carpet, and their noses are well off the ground. Children, however, habitually crawl and play on carpeted floors and are much more intimately exposed to any allergens or dirt they may contain.

It is foolish to deny that for many people carpet has many advantages in the home, including comfort and

ANTI-ALLERGY CARPET

This type of carpet is made from fibres containing antibacterial and antifungal agents. This has the effect of inhibiting mite growth, since mites cannot digest skin scales unless they are first broken down by bacteria and fungi. In theory, this should improve allergic symptoms. However, we do not know of any studies which support this. The carpet is more expensive than untreated types, and is available in a range of synthetic/wool mixes. The anti-mite effect should last for the life of the carpet, but you need to follow the maker's instructions for cleaning and care. Although the house-dust mite population is greatly reduced, the carpet should be vacuumed routinely with an HEPA-filter vacuum cleaner or central vacuum cleaner system to obtain maximum relief from house-dust mite allergens.

insulation against sound and loss of heat. If you do want some carpet in the home, short-pile carpets are easier to keep clean than deep-pile ones, or you may want to consider an anti-allergy carpet (*see box opposite*).

Choice of backing The foam backing of synthetic wall-to-wall carpets, especially those containing polyester, is usually finished with formaldehyde (*see p.69*), which will escape into the atmosphere at quite high levels for the first few months after being laid. If formaldehyde is a trigger for your allergic condition, choose carpeting that is backed with hessian or felt, instead of foam. All new foam-backed carpets should be aired well when they are first installed. Keeping the windows open whenever possible will help to prevent formalde-hyde gas building up.

Rugs and matting
Cotton rugs, including chenille, dhurrie (flat, woven, non-pile rugs), and rag rugs, can be used to add warmth and individuality, and to muffle noise. They are preferable to wall-to-wall carpet because house-dust mites and allergenic agents can be laundered out, but they need to be properly secured with rug grips or double-sided tape to make them safe to walk on. Ideally, cotton rugs should be colour-fast and machine-washable at a temperature of 56°C/133°F or above – the temperature needed to kill house-dust mites.

Wool rugs can be used, but they will need dry cleaning regularly to remove dust mites and allergens. Oriental wool rugs can last for generations, becoming family heirlooms. Dry steam cleaning (*see p. 93*) is an alternative to dry cleaning.

The durability of sisal, seagrass, and coir (coconut-husk fibre) rugs makes them a useful floor covering. However, they may harbour house-dust mites and so need thorough cleaning every few months. Alternatively, you can restrict their use to passageways and other heavily used areas of the home to make the most of their hardwearing features without compromising mite control too much.

Between launderings or dry cleaning, rugs and matting should be vacuumed regularly (daily or weekly, depending on how much foot traffic they receive), ideally with a HEPA-filtered vacuum cleaner or central vacuum system (*see pp. 74–5*).

Hard-surface flooring
Although a few people argue that removing carpets is not wise, since they trap large quantities of dust that would, otherwise, be circulating freely in the air, experts in general advise hard-surface flooring as a healthier alternative. A simple cleaning routine will ensure dust does not accumulate.

If you decide to retain the comfort factor and have a fitted carpet in the living or family rooms, then still consider taking carpets and non-washable rugs out of children's bedrooms, since children spend so much time sleeping or playing in their rooms.

Choice of materials There are several choices of hard-surface flooring available, including hardwood, linoleum, vinyl, and ceramic tiles.

Ceramic tiles are particularly suitable for the "wet" rooms of the home – the kitchen and bathroom – while linoleum and vinyl flooring, which is available in an extremely wide range of colours and designs, can be installed successfully in any room. If linoleum or vinyl is used in bathrooms and kitchens, however, you will have to wipe up any water spills quickly to stop moisture working its way underneath the material. Cork is another option, but there is the possibility of it becoming colonized by mites. This is less likely if sealed cork is used.

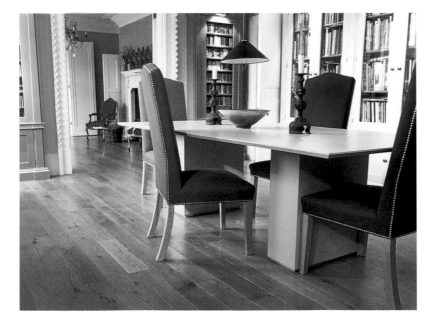

Hard-surface flooring, including laminated or solid wood, is the preferred option for a low-allergen home. Avoid grooved wood surfaces – these become dust traps and are then difficult to keep clean.

Hardwood floors should be sealed if used in a kitchen or bathroom to prevent water penetration.

Hardwood Modern hardwood flooring is often available as a laminated material – a thin hardwood layer is glued to a plywood or other artificial wooden base. It is nearly always prestained and prefinished. In general, water-based adhesives, stains, and other finishes give off less odour and "out-gas" (*see pp. 68–9*) less than solvent-based finishes. Laminated floors are cheaper than solid-wood floors, but they cannot be sanded down later or refinished as real wood

can. Solid-wood flooring comprises planks or parquet (patterned blocks).

Linoleum or vinyl Due to its low cost, ease of installation, and the wide range of patterns and colours available, vinyl and linoleum flooring is very popular. Vinyl flooring is made from vinyl plastic, primarily polyvinyl chloride (PVC). When new, it out-gases high levels of chemicals, particularly plasticizers. Although linoleum is made from natural ingredients, it is based on linseed oil, which, when new, gives off a powerful odour that may cause respiratory irritation. If you are fitting

either of these materials, open windows and thoroughly air the room until the smell has completely disappeared. This should not take more than a few days.

Ceramic tiling There are various types of ceramic tiles to choose from, with mosaic, quarry, glazed, and slate tiles being popular. These are available in sizes, colours, and surface textures to suit most styles and situations. Glazed or vitreous tiles have an impervious surface and do not need to be sealed. Porous, unsealed tiles may harbour bacteria and other microorganisms and easily become stained. To make cleaning easier porous tiles should always be sealed when used in kitchens and bathrooms.

The grouting between tiles can harbour mould if it becomes cracked or is constantly damp. Most common allergenic moulds prefer an acidic environment, so it is best to choose a grouting that is strongly alkaline in its chemical composition.

Wall coverings and windows

There are many forms of wall covering, ranging from wallpaper to wood panelling, although some are better than others for the low-allergen home.

Wallpaper This is a very popular method of decorating walls. It instantly changes the "feel" of a room and literally papers over minor defects in the surface of less-than-perfect walls. Smooth, washable wallpaper is preferable, since textured wallpaper is more prone to trapping dust. Damp is

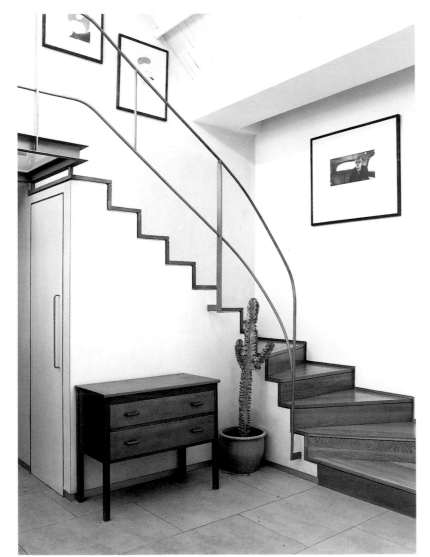

In this hallway, the lack of clutter and the streamlined walls, floors, and other surfaces minimize the places where dust can collect, so making the area easy to keep clean.

unlikely to be a problem behind the wallpaper unless the wall itself is cold enough to encourage condensation. Most wallpaper glues contain fungicides, which inhibit the growth of mould. If you are allergic to mould, beware of mould patches and the release of mould spores when you are stripping off old wallpaper. Some people develop allergic dermatitis when in contact with the carboxymethylcellulose that is found in some wallpaper pastes, and so you should wear protective gloves if you are sensitive to this substance.

Paint   For the low-allergen home, paint is the recommended option for walls. The range of paint colours is so wide that there is bound to be exactly the right shade, and if a flat colour is not to your taste then you can always try your hand at stencilling, wood-graining, or one of the many other decorative paint effects. It is worthwhile giving some thought to your choice of brand, however, since the solvents contained in some paints can provoke symptoms in those with allergies (see pp. 66–7).

Wall panelling   Wooden panelling has undergone a popular revival recently with the renewed interest in the American Shaker style of decoration and in the decorative styles of the Victorian era. Unfortunately, wall panelling in the form of a veneer over particle board, plywood, or hardboard is usually made with glues that emit formaldehyde, and therefore cannot be recommended for the low-allergen home (see pp. 70–1).

Windows   Your choice of window dressing impacts on allergen levels. Heavy curtains are not recommended because they collect dust and are hard

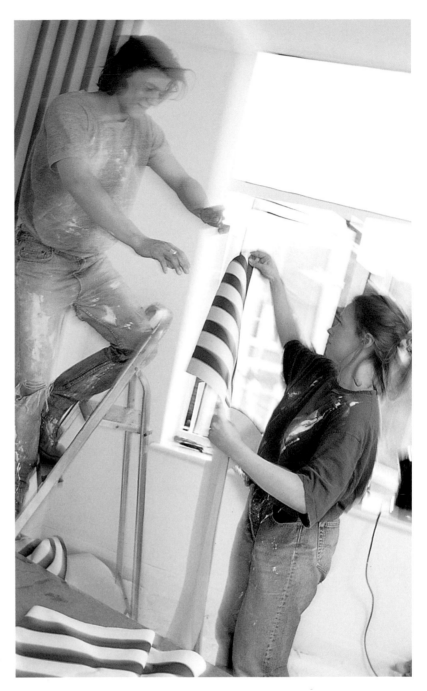

to keep clean. They may also act as a place for dust mites to breed. Easily cleaned blinds (shades) are the preferred option, especially plastic or wooden slatted types. Vertical blinds collect less dust and are easier to clean than horizontal ones, but easy-clean roller blinds can also be satisfactory.

Double-glazing (secondary glazing) prevents or reduces condensation, so reducing the potential for mould

Areas of damp trapped behind wallpaper may lead to the onset of mould. However, most modern wallpaper glues contain fungicides which inhibit the growth of mould.

growth. Modern units also have trickle ventilators – a sliding control in the frame to allow in a little air while the window remains shut – to provide background ventilation and help reduce humidity, which also helps to inhibit mite populations and mould.

Home Improvements

Before the 1960s, a long working week and few holidays were the rule for most people. Leisure time and activities were limited. Within a generation, this has changed. The modern family has more leisure time and more money to spend. One of the most popular leisure activities is the home – maintaining it, decorating it, improving it.

Many home-improvement products have been developed to meet consumer demand. These include modern paints, glues, and varnishes – and organic solvents, such as white spirit (mineral spirit), are important ingredients of many of them. In general, these solvents evaporate quickly once exposed to air and are, therefore, known as volatile organic compounds, or VOCs (*see also pp. 68–9*).

Paints and varnishes

The fumes given off as solvents from paints and varnishes can act as an irritant – especially for those with rhinitis or asthma – causing symptoms that include watery eyes, sneezing, or coughing. In some cases, these irritants may even trigger an asthma attack. As a general rule, the higher a product's VOC content, the stronger its odour.

Solvent (VOC) content Paints are either oil or water based. Most paints used for walls are water based, while those used for woodwork could be either oil or water based. Oil-based paints are much more likely to cause problems for people with allergies, however, because they contain high concentrations of solvent. The solvent

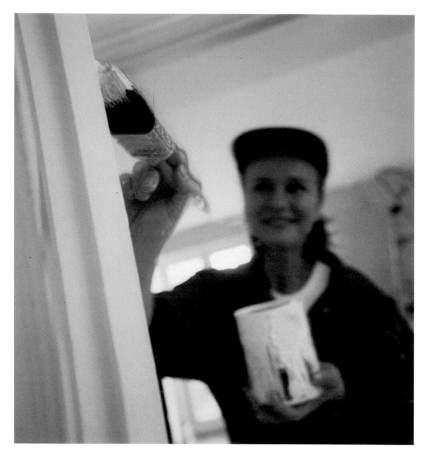

is used to thin the oil, which, in turn, makes the paint easy to apply. Surprisingly, some oil paints may contain more than 50 percent solvent.

As the paint dries, the solvents evaporate into the air, initially at high concentrations, and this may provoke an irritant reaction. Water-based paints and varnishes do not contain such high concentrations of solvents.

Major paint manufacturers advise people with respiratory allergies to use water-based paints and varnishes for walls and woodwork. These are usually low-odour and dry more quickly than oil-based paints.

Water-based products are also promoted for exterior use, but paints

Water-based paint has less odour than oil-based types due to the reduced solvent content. Even so, make sure that there is proper ventilation where you are working. Use the chart (see right) as a guide to alternative paints.

and similar products are unlikely to trigger symptoms when used outside.

Alternative paints With some people with allergies, even water-based paints may provoke symptoms; others may simply want to minimize their overall exposure to VOCs. While they are not as readily available as paints from the major manufacturers, specialist companies generally provide a good range of allergen-friendly products (*see opposite*).

A guide to alternative paint products

Composition	Advantages	Disadvantages
Protein based (based on casein, milk products, bone, or glue)	● No VOCs ● Odourless/low odour ● Non-allergenic	● Moisture-sensitive ● Suitable for interior use only ● Not washable ● Matte finish only ● No glosses, varnishes, or wood paints available
Resin based (based on wood resin and vegetable oil)	● Pleasant smell ● Wide range of paints and varnishes ● Durable ● Washable	● Solvent based, using a solvent which may be potentially irritant, such as turpentine and white spirit (mineral spirit) ● Requires good ventilation
Resin based (synthetic resins)	● Wide range of varnishes and paints, including wood stains and gloss paints ● Low odour or odourless ● VOC-free ● Washable ● Durable ● Non-allergenic	● Composed of synthetic resins, which are, however, free of vinyl chloride (a substance that can be harmful to the environment)
Lime based (limewash based on lime plus animal or vegetable fats)	● Non-allergenic	● Dusty, soft film when dry ● Not washable or of limited washability ● Matte finish only ● No glosses, varnishes, or wood paints
Stone paint (based on silicate)	● Highly durable ● Washable ● Inherently anti-fungal/algal ● Non-allergenic	● Matte finish only ● No gloss paints or varnishes ● Normally used only on exteriors ● Rubs off against clothing ● Alkaline (protect skin and eyes) ● Very high energy input at raw-material stage
Oil-bound emulsions (latex paints based on vegetable oil)	● Washable ● Fairly durable in interiors ● Generally non-allergenic	● May contain VOCs ● Yellows with age ● Best used as interior finish only ● Usually matte finish only ● Paint may separate in the can ● May be allergenic

Wood preservatives

There are numerous products for protecting wood from insect or fungal attack. Many are solvent-based, however, and potentially dangerous for those with allergies. Handle these chemicals carefully to avoid skin contact and avoid breathing in the fumes. Wood preservatives may cause irritation of the skin and mucous membranes, as well as headaches, dizziness, and nausea.

Whenever possible, buy water-based wood preservatives. These contain much lower levels of VOCs than standard types and smell less strongly, and may also be less irritating for people with respiratory conditions.

VOLATILE ORGANIC COMPOUNDS

These compounds, commonly referred to as VOCs, are one of the main home pollutants. They contain carbon, hence the term "organic", and the ease with which they evaporate at room temperature makes them "volatile".

There has been much discussion about the health effects of VOCs, which are found in many domestic products. Although many experts recommend that VOC levels should be kept low inside the home, there is still debate on precisely what are safe levels for many of these substances. VOCs are not allergens, but they may act as irritants in some people with allergies, provoking symptoms such as sneezing, watery eyes, a "tight" chest, or wheeziness. For the vast majority VOCs cause little problem.

Sources of VOCs

Most VOCs are synthetic and are derived from petrochemicals. They are found in many home-improvement and cleaning products. A few, however, occur naturally; for example, the citrus fragrance of an orange or the eye-stinging vapour given off by an onion when you cut into it.

The evaporation of VOCs into the air (known as "out-gassing") may occur rapidly and disperse quickly, as when you cut into an orange, or it may occur slowly over many months from products such as board-based furniture. This slow leakage helps to contribute to the background level of VOCs found within the typical home.

Common sources of domestic VOCs

Domestic sources	Comments	Remedies
Paints and varnishes	Ordinary paints, particularly gloss types, often have strong odours and emit high levels of VOCs while drying. Many paints contain formaldehyde in the form of preservatives, which will continue to out-gas once the paint is dry. Nearly all commonly available paint strippers are solvent-based and potentially irritating.	Make sure that the area being painted is well ventilated and keep it ventilated until the smell disperses. Or choose low-odour or environmentally friendly paints. Check the type of preservative included. There are water-based polyurethane varnishes and paint strippers available, which give off less odour.
Wood preservatives	These are highly toxic substances often dissolved in organic solvents.	Restrict their use to confirmed outbreaks of woodworm and decay. Choose water-based products, which give off less odour.
Adhesives	Many of these products release VOCs and other irritant substances during use.	Consider water-based products, as these will contain (and release) less solvent. Provide good ventilation during use.
Cleaning products	Many of these products release VOCs and other irritant substances during use.	Rediscover the cleaning materials of earlier times. They are the basis of many commercial brands and are often cheaper and safer to use (see pp. 76–7).
Board-based furniture and flooring boards	The glues used in particle board contain the VOC formaldehyde. Furniture or flooring made with this board can out-gas for up to several years.	Consider solid wood for cabinets and shelving. Low-emission flooring boards may be available. Seal in formaldehyde on exposed board with paint or varnish, or choose plastic-laminated board.
Insulation	Urea-formaldehyde foam (UFFI) was once commonly used as insulation.	This is a long-term source of formaldehyde. Use an alternative (see p. 109).

Reducing VOC levels

The first and most crucial step is to make sure that your home is well ventilated, as this will prevent VOC levels building up in the air you breathe. If you still think that VOCs from particular products are irritating your allergic symptoms, then try to avoid the products responsible, or look for alternatives (see below).

Formaldehyde in the home

This substance is a common VOC. It has attracted much attention recently because of the controversy concerning its health effects. Low concentrations in the air may irritate the eyes, nose, and throat, particularly in people with rhinitis or asthma, and may cause running eyes, sneezing, and coughing.

Formaldehyde is found in minute quantities in numerous household products, but most contain too little to cause any problems for the vast majority of people with allergies. However, a few domestic products contain formaldehyde in high concentrations. These products out-gas for months, sometimes years, even though this may be at very low levels:

- Board-based wood products, widely used for flooring, shelving, and especially flat-packed kit furniture (see p. 71)
- Foam-backed carpets and underlay (see pp. 62–3)
- Paint preservatives (see pp. 66–7)

Bear in mind that the amount of formaldehyde emitted from all products decreases with time, and that after a few weeks to months it should be at extremely low levels and very unlikely to cause any problems for most people with allergies.

Domestic sources	Comments	Remedies
New carpets and some floorings	The "new" smell of carpets and vinyl flooring is caused by VOCs out-gassing from these products.	Ventilate new carpets and vinyl flooring until the smell disappears and the amount of VOCs given off is greatly reduced. Consider using hard-surface flooring instead.
Hygiene and personal-care products	Fragrances used in perfumes and cosmetics may provoke symptoms, such as sneezing and wheezing, in some people with allergies, as well as causing skin irritation.	Use non-scented and hypo-allergenic products (see pp. 77, 84, and 103).
Art and hobby materials	Many contain solvents causing irritation when they come into skin contact or are inhaled.	Use in a well-ventilated area or choose water-based products instead.
Aerosols	These release high concentrations of VOCs, provoking respiratory symptoms in some people with allergies.	Use in a well-ventilated area, well away from anybody with asthma. If possible, choose non-aerosol products.
Air fresheners	Propellants and preservatives used in pressurized air fresheners may act as an irritant in respiratory allergies.	Good ventilation minimizes odours, as will an air-filtering unit (see p. 58). Use natural products for odour absorption (see p. 85).
Dry-cleaned garments	Some of the chemicals used in the dry-cleaning process are highly irritant.	Air dry-cleaned garments outside until all the smell has gone.
Non-iron, easy-care, or crease-resistant fabrics	If you see these descriptions on clothes' labels and articles of bedding, they indicate that the fabrics have been treated with a finish containing formaldehyde.	A few people have reported sensitivity to the formaldehyde content of some of the treatments used for clothing and bedding. Natural untreated fabrics, such as unbleached cotton, are available from specialist suppliers.

Furnishings and Fixtures

Choosing furnishings and fixtures for the home is a very individual affair, but more than personal taste is involved – your choice affects the level of allergens and irritants in the home.

Soft furnishings

Leather or vinyl is the preferred covering for soft furnishings, as dust mites find it inhospitable, while fabric-upholstered furniture provides the ideal home for dust mites. Consider replacing fabric upholstery with leather or vinyl, or other hard-surface materials, such as wood or plastic – or

at least reduce the number of soft furnishings you have in your home.

Leather or vinyl only needs wiping over with a damp cloth weekly to keep it clean of dust and mites, while controlling mites in fabric-upholstered furnishings is far more difficult. Several approaches are used to try to do this, or to neutralize or remove the allergen, and these also apply to other mite reservoirs, such as carpets.

Acaricides These mite-killing chemicals penetrate only the uppermost layers of fabric, so mites deeper down

survive – and the mite allergen still needs to be removed afterwards by vacuuming. The most-researched acaricide, benzyl benzoate, may persist for up to a year after application, although most studies suggest it should be reapplied several times a year. One study suggests acaricides may reduce symptoms of mite-related rhinitis, but there is a lack of evidence that they are generally beneficial. As no long-term safety studies have been done in the home, you may not want to use acaricides in children's rooms.

Denaturing agent Tannic acid alters the structure of all allergens, (denatures them) including pollen and dander, as well as mite allergen, so that they no longer cause an allergic reaction. It needs applying three to four times a year, but may discolour pale fabrics or carpets. It is probably harmless to people and animals.

Steam treatment Mites near the surface are killed by steam, although those deeper down in soft furnishings (and mattresses) are likely to be unaffected. Ask for independent proof that the steam treatment is sufficiently hot for long enough to denature mite allergen, as not all steam treatments achieve this. The dead mites and allergen are removed afterwards by vacuuming. Steam cleaning probably needs to be done every three months.

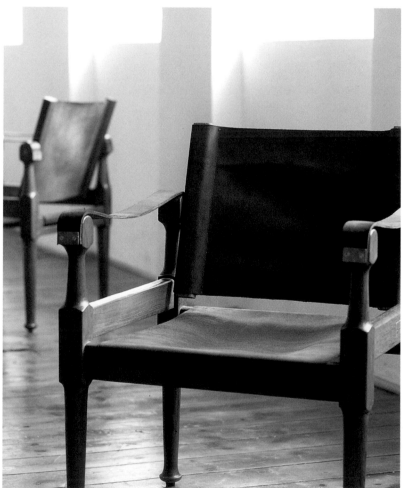

Wooden furniture, simply made, with the minimum of detailing where dust can collect, and upholstered in leather, makes the management of dust-mite allergy far easier.

Vacuuming Domestic vacuum cleaners, even HEPA-filtered models, are not powerful enough to clean fabric-covered furnishings sufficiently of mites, which cling to the fabric, or of mite allergen to justify the effort involved.

Heat treatment This treatment kills mites and denatures mite allergen. The whole sofa, couch, or chair, slightly dampened with a tannic acid solution, is heated to about 100°C/212°F inside a tent-like envelope. Contractors recommend annual treatment. It is also suitable for mattresses, bedding, soft cushions, and curtains.

Liquid nitrogen This freezes mites to death and loosens the allergen-containing dirt, which can then be removed with a vacuum cleaner. It must be applied by a contractor once or twice a year. It does not leave chemical residues and is safe.

Board-based furniture

Various forms of "board" – an inexpensive wood-based product – include laminated board, chipboard (particle board), hardboard, and medium-density fibreboard (MDF). It is often used in flooring, roofing, shelving, and furniture, and is composed of wood components bonded with glue or resin made with formaldehyde. Some,

> **TIP**
>
> When using board for home improvements, make sure your work area is well ventilated. Work outside if at all possible and wear a dust respirator face mask while sawing the material. Consider airing the board outside, under cover, for at least a week before working with it, and use paint or varnish to seal in as much of the formaldehyde as possible.

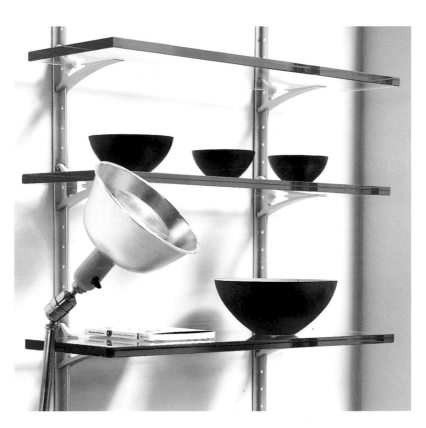

such as MDF, contain much higher levels of formaldehyde than others. The glue or resin gives off (out-gases) formaldehyde, a colourless, pungent gas. Some people with rhinitis or asthma find that formaldehyde worsens their allergic symptoms. The amount of formaldehyde out-gassed is greatest when the board is new, in the first few weeks to several months, but then gradually decreases.

Choosing new furniture

Nearly all modern, mass-produced wood furniture, even that labelled "solid wood", contains some board. This includes veneered furniture, in which a layer of fine wood covers a less-expensive board carcass.

When buying new board-based furniture, including kitchen or bathroom cabinets, try to choose furniture made from board encased in a plastic laminate, which has the effect of minimizing formaldehyde emission. You may

Metal brackets and glass shelving make a stylish addition to a room, providing an opportunity for unusual lighting effects, but ideally shelves should be behind glass doors to stop dust collecting.

want to consider airing new products for a week or two, in a dry place under cover so that they do not warp, to make sure the peak period for formaldehyde out-gassing has passed.

Look for exposed areas of board where the laminate has not covered the carcass; these are the areas where formaldehyde will most readily out-gas. Painting any exposed board with several layers of paint or varnish is said by some people to minimize the emission of formaldehyde gas.

Because of the formaldehyde issue, you may want to consider using as much solid wood furniture as possible, despite its extra expense. Softwood, metal, or glass can all be used for shelving. A few people find that the terpene vapours given off by soft-woods worsen allergic symptoms.

Cleaning Your Home

Run your finger along a dusty surface in your home and the light gray powder on your fingertip will consist mainly of dead skin scales. These are shed from the human body as the skin continually renews itself. Along with skin scales, dust also contains fibres, particles of pollution, pollen, animal dander (skin scales and saliva), and microorganisms, such as mould spores, bacteria, and, of course, the ubiquitous house-dust mite with its allergenic fecal droppings.

Because dust is composed mainly of skin scales (the dust mite's favourite food) it tends to accumulate in the most heavily used parts of the home, especially in beds, carpets, and furniture upholstered in fabric. These places also trap humidity and warmth, providing the ideal breeding environment for these tiny creatures.

Dust is, therefore, a potent source of allergens, especially of mite allergens, but also, to a lesser extent, of pollen, mould, and animal allergens. For those individuals who are sensitive to mite allergen, a dusty home is likely to be a significant factor in their allergic condition.

While it is likely that the stronger the sensitivity to mite allergen the more effective dust-avoidance and mite-elimination measures are likely to be, dust-mite allergen is not the only cause of allergic symptoms. Therefore, it is important to consult your doctor before buying products aimed specifically at reducing dust-mite allergen – for example, HEPA filter vacuum cleaners (see pp. 74–5) or anti-mite barrier covers for beds and bed linen (see pp. 82–3).

The amount of effort you need to put into removing dust from your home depends on the severity of the allergic symptoms you experience. Being realistic, however, most of us have only limited time to spend on cleaning, so it is best to concentrate your efforts on the rooms most used by the allergy sufferer. In general, the bedroom is the most important room to keep free of dust mites and dust.

Reducing clutter

One of the most important allergy-reducing steps you can take is to rid your home of clutter. The simple truth is that clutter collects dust, so resolve to stop giving space to all those objects, curios, or knick-knacks you do not truly cherish. Take your time and go through your home, room by room. Aim to keep surfaces clear of clutter so that you can easily wipe away the dust that does settle there. Those objects you decide to keep can be placed in display cabinets – even books can be kept on glass-fronted shelves. Rid your home of unwanted larger items, too, such as that easy chair you have never really liked or those cushions on the sofa you always push aside before sitting down.

Dusting

Avoid using a feather duster. Rather than removing dust, all it does is flick it up into the air where it can be breathed in or cause problems by settling on the eyes or on the mucous membranes of the nose. Dust can remain airborne for several hours before settling down once again, all the time posing problems for those sensitive to house-dust allergen. Instead, it is better to damp-dust using a slightly damp, but not wet, cloth. Dust-attracting (electrostatic) cloths are also available, or you may prefer to clean surfaces using a vacuum cleaner fitted with a suitable attachment.

Uncluttered surfaces are much easier to keep clean of dust, which contains allergens, such as mite droppings, mould spores, and pollen, and contaminants, such as pollution particulates.

ROOM MAKE-OVER

If you are thinking of redecorating a room or buying new furniture and accessories for the home, consider the following points:

- Will the room be easy to dust? Simple, uncluttered designs collect less dust and are easier to keep clean than complicated, fussy ones. This applies to anything from bed headboards and curtains to shelving, ornaments, and lighting.
- If you are replacing a carpet, consider putting down a hard-surface flooring material with washable cotton rugs. Carpets are a major reservoir of dust mites and sometimes moulds, too.
- It is not just horizontal surfaces that collect dust – walls, too, can harbour dust. In the light of this, choose wipable paint or non-textured wallpaper.
- Avoid ornate mouldings, skirting (base) boards, and lighting units.
- The tops of cabinets and open shelves are notorious dust traps, so build cabinets right up to the ceiling and put doors on shelves.

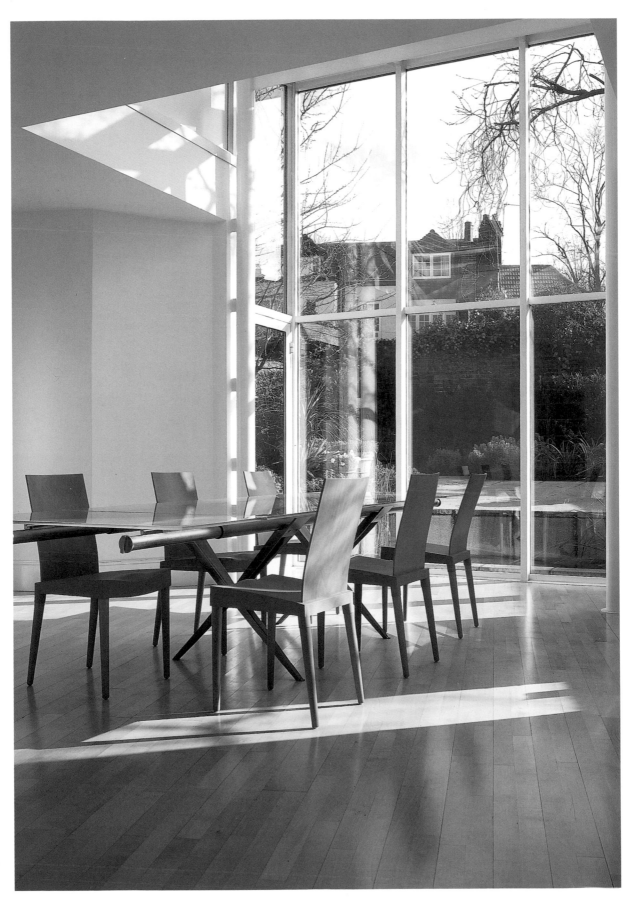

VACUUM CLEANERS

Vacuuming is important, but it can only help as part of a planned mite-reduction programme. If you decide to retain carpets and soft furnishings, as well as curtains or drapes and unprotected mattresses, you will have to vacuum daily in order to keep the mites in check. Even with this effort, vacuuming alone is not enough to reduce allergic symptoms. Other measures, especially the use of anti-mite barrier covers for bedding (see pp. 82–3), are also necessary.

Many families prefer to remove all carpeting and to use furniture that mites cannot colonize, such as wood, leather, or vinyl. These measures, combined with regular vacuuming, can make a real difference.

There are two main types of vacuum cleaning equipment available: freestanding or portable appliances and central vacuum systems. Some freestanding cleaners use bags to collect the dust, while others are bagless and deposit the dust in a

canister that needs to be emptied on a regular basis.

Vacuum cleaners stir up some dust when in use, and you may wish to wear a dust mask if you develop allergic symptoms (such as sneezing or chest tightness) when vacuuming.

Conventional vacuum cleaners

Vacuum cleaners usually suck air through a standard filter bag before pumping it back into the room. The bag collects only the largest particles of dust, allowing the rest, including allergens, back into the room.

Higher-grade filter bags can be used instead of standard types. These are available for many brands of cleaner and they do trap small dust particles more effectively. However, unless they are HEPA filters, which can filter out mite allergen and cat dander, they will not be effective for all allergic conditions. Check first that your standard vacuum cleaner is powerful enough to suck air through the close-set fibres of the HEPA filter bag.

HEPA-filter vacuum cleaners

Many modern vacuum cleaners are now fitted with HEPA (high-efficiency particulate air) filters – special filters that capture almost 100 percent of mite allergen, pollen, and cat dander – most of which are suitable for people with allergies. Some of these models are expensive, so seek advice from your doctor, allergy association, or consumer organization before deciding

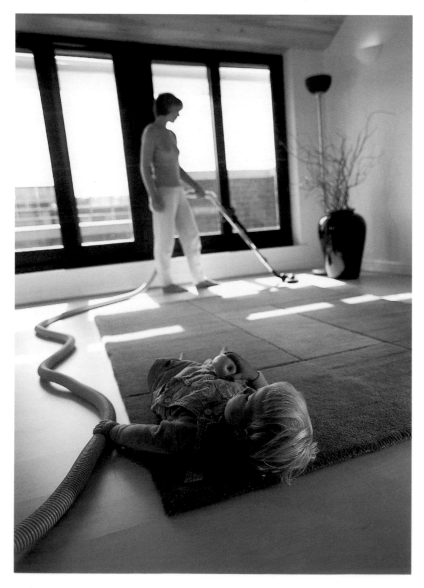

The lightweight hose of a central vacuum cleaner is plugged through wall sockets into hidden ducting, down which all the dust is sucked to a large, external receptacle.

CHOOSING AND USING A VACUUM CLEANER

- Never vacuum just before bedtime – any dust disturbed will be breathed in as you sleep.
- Check independent reports to make sure that the cleaner is able to collect large quantities of dust and retain it without blowing any of it back into the room.
- The dust must be collected in a receptacle that can be emptied without causing problems for the allergy sufferer.
- Make sure the machine is easy to move around and lift.
- Check with independent consumer groups and organizations or an allergy association if they recommend particular brands.
- Remember to add in the cost of replacement filters.
- Make sure that the machine is powerful enough to clean surface dirt from upholstery. The higher the wattage, the more powerful the suction, and the more dirt it can collect. However, it is difficult to remove mites effectively from fabric even with powerful cleaners.
- Useful features include: automatic floor selection (adjusts for different heights of carpet and flooring types) or interchangeable heads, variable suction power for different materials (for curtains or rugs), and a turbo head (good for cut-pile carpets).

on the model most suitable for you. Even HEPA-filter vacuum cleaners stir up some dust when in use, but the suction around the outside edge of their brushes produce far fewer airborne particles compared to the amount thrown up by conventional cleaners. In addition, revolving brushes (as used in a "turbo head") are more effective at collecting allergens from cut-pile carpets.

Cyclonic vacuum cleaners

These bagless machines use a centrifugal airflow to collect dust and deposit it in a canister. The cleaners also use HEPA filters that do not let dust pass back into the room. But since they do not seal the dust away, as do filter-bag machines, it can be difficult to empty the canister without breathing in the dust or getting some of it on your clothes and skin.

Water-filter vacuum cleaners

These machines suck the dust-laden air through a water reservoir, where water-soluble dust, including allergens,

is left behind in the water. There is concern that some brands of cleaner emit dust particles in the form of an aerosolized spray, and that the water reservoir itself may become contaminated with mould unless it is emptied and thoroughly dried after each use.

Central vacuum cleaners

A cleaning system of this type, which is a popular feature in some countries, consists of a suction unit and dust-collecting bag or bin placed in a basement, utility room, garage, or understairs closet. To use the system, you plug a long, flexible hose into strategically placed sockets, and the dust is transported via narrow ducting hidden in the building's structure to the collecting bag or bin. Because the motor unit and dust receptacle are stationary, they can be far larger and

The design of some vacuum-cleaner dust-collection bags means that they seal up the dust and allergens, making them safe for an allergic person to handle.

provide more powerful suction than any portable cleaner.

Central vacuum cleaners are easy to maintain and operate, especially since a lightweight hose is all you need to carry around your home. The collecting bag or bin of domestic units needs emptying about every 6 to 12 months – although an allergy sufferer should avoid doing this.

Most central vacuum cleaners are vented to the outdoors. Outdoor-vented cleaners are preferable for those with allergies, as the air pulled into the vacuum cleaner will then go straight outside, so eliminating any concern that undesirable allergens can escape back into the living space.

Central vacuum cleaners can be fitted into a home quite easily after it has been built. Rather than being run up inside the walls, the ducting that connects the sockets is usually run up inside a cupboard (often an under-stairs cupboard). Only two sockets are needed for most homes (one upstairs and one downstairs) because of the length (about 30m/98ft) of the hose which can normally stretch the length of the house if the sockets are placed in the centre of the home.

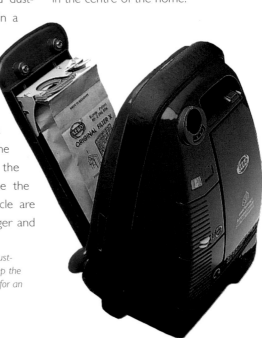

CLEANING PRODUCTS

Many commonly available cleaners – especially aerosol products, such as furniture sprays, which disperse a fine spray into the air – give off solvents or other chemicals that may provoke symptoms in people with respiratory allergies. Many products also have irritant fragrances that sensitive people need to avoid.

People with skin contact allergies may find many different products irritating, and need to take care to protect their hands whenever they use cleaning materials. Those who have had childhood eczema are much more likely to develop irritant hand dermatitis, although anybody could develop problems if they are exposed to certain substances for long enough. It is common, for example, for new parents to develop irritant hand dermatitis, since once the baby is at home the

GLOVES FOR HAND CARE

Whether you have sensitive skin or not, always wear protective gloves when using substances containing potential irritants, such as detergents and cleaning products. Bear in mind that contact irritant dermatitis can develop in anyone with continued exposure. Household rubber gloves are normally made of latex and can be lined with either a cotton flock or a smooth lining. A few people are allergic to the latex that is present in the gloves (see pp. 22–3) or in the powder inside the glove that makes it easier to put the glove on. Special gloves for latex-sensitive people are available. People with sensitive skin should use very lightweight polythene gloves, as used by hairdressers, to wash their hair.

parents come into contact with strong chemicals – such as sterilizing fluids or diaper-soaking solutions – if they don't protect their hands.

Household cleaners

Don't assume that cleaning-product labels such as "eco-safe" or "environmentally friendly" mean that the contents are necessarily suitable for allergy sufferers. These terms may simply indicate that the packaging is recyclable or biodegradable, or that the contents are concentrated (so less packaging is required).

In a reaction against chemical-based household products, there is growing interest in traditional methods of cleaning using such materials as baking soda, table salt, and vinegar (see Bibliography, p. 138). As an example, a safe method of oven cleaning is to sprinkle spillages with water and then add baking soda and more water. Leave overnight and wipe away the next morning, using a mild abrasive pad if necessary. Then wash over with some liquid soap and rinse.

Clothes cleaning

For people with allergies, there are two main considerations when it comes to doing the laundry. The first concerns symptoms (respiratory or skin) that are made worse by contact with mite allergen; the second concerns eczema, dermatitis, or urticaria that is caused or made worse by some washing products.

House-dust mites can survive washing temperatures up to 56°C/133°F. Although the mite allergen will be washed out at lower temperatures, the mites themselves will cling to the

fabric using suckers on their feet. This is why all bed linen (sheets, pillow cases, duvet covers, and so on) should be made of cotton, which is washable at the temperatures needed to kill the mites outright.

Alternatively, you can add a dilute benzyl benzoate solution to a lower-temperature wash water used for bed linen. The benzyl benzoate kills mites, which are then washed out along with the allergen. Make sure that you follow the manufacturer's recommendations regarding quantities to use.

Benzyl benzoate is generally considered to be safe, but little is known about its effects when used long-term as an acaricide. If you do use it for cleaning bed linen or clothes, you may want to program your washing machine to give extra rinses. Alternatively, you could replace your bed linen with cotton items and reserve the benzyl benzoate for use with items, such as curtains, that are not in constant, close skin contact.

By a process of trial and error most allergic people discover which washing product best suits their skin condition. Whichever it is, try not to use too much, and rinse thoroughly to avoid any potentially irritating residues. If you are experimenting with different products to discover which ones are suitable, remember to rinse your washing machine out thoroughly to remove all traces of the previous one. It is also wise to try any new product on just one or two items first, particularly if the allergic person has very sensitive skin.

Biological washing products contain enzymes to break down proteins, such as milk or blood, that cause stains.

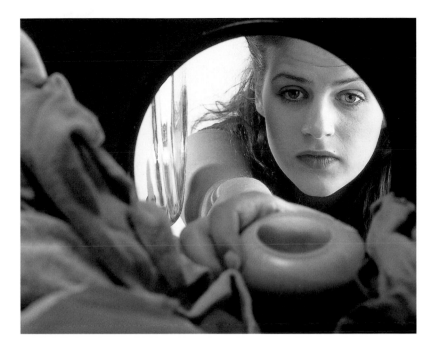

Some emollients used for eczema leave a greasy film that may rot the rubber seals of washing machines. Run the machine empty on a hot wash with a cupful of baking soda to remove it.

occur, try using one tablespoon of washing soda, sodium bicarbonate, or borax per washing load. Another option is a laundry ball, a chemical-free alternative to detergents.

A few people with eczema can tolerate fabric conditioners, but many sufferers find that the perfume they contain irritates their condition. If this is the case, use a quarter cup of baking soda, vinegar, or borax instead.

Many brands of stain remover contain solvent-type irritant chemicals – often indicated by the manufacturer's precautions concerning their use. In addition, they are often highly fragranced. Simple home-made stain removers, based on vinegar, club soda, or corn starch, can be just as effective as these stronger commercial brands.

People with eczema may find that their skin condition is made worse by exposure to these enzymes (which may also cause respiratory symptoms), and often find non-biological products more acceptable. However, if these also cause irritation, then products labelled as suitable for "sensitive skin" may be a better option, or you could even try old-fashioned soap flakes. Sensitivity to every type of washing product is rare, but if this should

LOOKING AFTER YOUR HANDS

For people with eczema or dermatitis, the hands are one of the commonest sites to be affected. Here are some simple steps to take to protect your hands from exposure to irritants.

Hand washing
- Wash your hands only when necessary – too much hand washing is generally bad for the skin.
- Use lukewarm water with a soap substitute. Ask your doctor to prescribe one or ask the pharmacist for suggestions.
- Always rinse thoroughly to remove any irritant residues.
- Dry between your fingers as this is where the skin is very prone to dryness and cracking.
- Wear household rubber gloves with a pair of cotton liners when washing up – latex-free ones if you are latex-sensitive.

Detergents and cleaning agents
- Try to avoid direct contact with these products. Keep the outside of packages clear of content spills.
- Wash your hands under running water if contact is made.
- Use non-biological laundry products.
- Never use too much powder or liquid.
- Avoid perfumed fabric conditioners.

Polishes
- Avoid direct contact with metal, wax, shoe, floor, furniture, and window polishes.
- Wear rubber gloves – latex-free if necessary – or cotton gloves.

Solvents and stain removers
- Avoid skin contact with white spirit (mineral spirit), trichloroethylene, petrol, turpentine, and thinners.
- If contact is made, wash your hands in lukewarm water using a little soap.

Fruit and vegetables
- Do not peel any citrus fruit, onions or garlic with your bare hands.
- Be careful when handling food – some people with eczema experience a burning sensation or itching when handling foods to which they are allergic. The juice from fruits and vegetables may act as allergens or irritants. For example, some people sneeze when peeling potatoes, although they can eat them when cooked without problems.

Rings
- Contact dermatitis can often be caused by rings, especially if they contain nickel.
- Clean rings with a brush when they are dirty and leave overnight in a weak solution of ammonia. Rinse thoroughly in the morning.

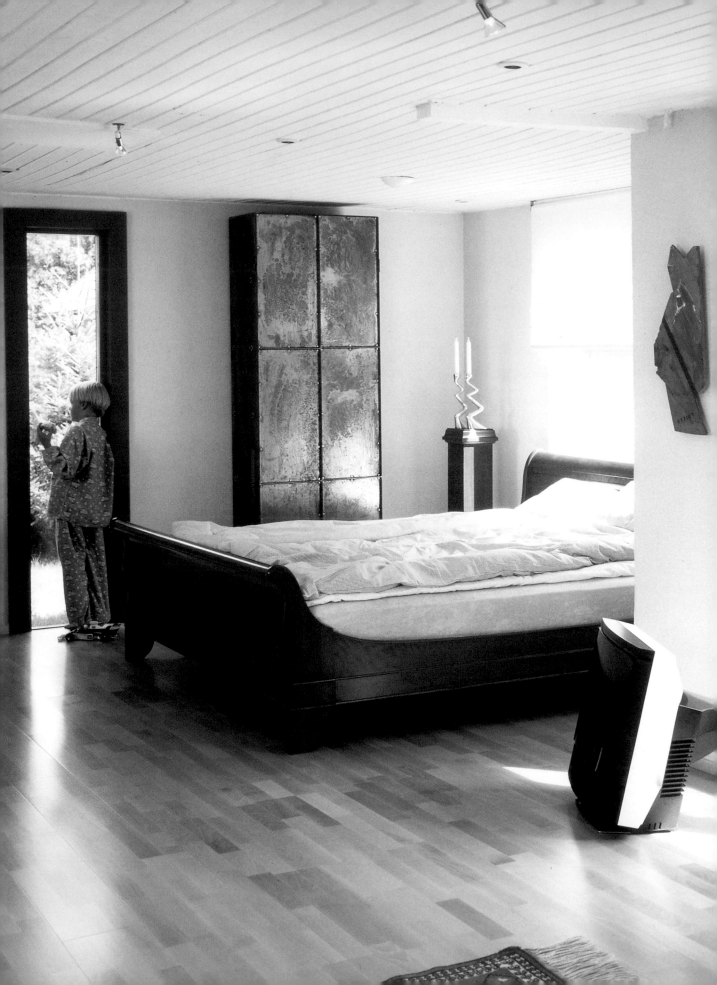

The Ideal Room

The question that people with allergic conditions most often ask health professionals is: "What can I do to improve my condition and so reduce my dependency on regular medication?" Assuming that tests show you are allergic to factors in the home environment, the answer is to modify your home to decrease your exposure to the major interior allergens and irritants. While this advice is easy to give, there is in fact a dearth of practical guidance on just how to go about doing this. In the following pages, you will find down-to-earth advice on what you can do to help bring about relief from allergic symptoms.

After reading this advice through, don't wear yourself, or your pocket, out making changes in a hurry. Take time to think through your own or your family's symptoms, what you might be reacting to in your home, and how serious the reaction is. Unless you have a major problem, make small changes first, and slowly.

Start with the easier and inexpensive steps to see if they improve your symptoms. Don't make the mistake of trying to do everything you might want to at once. Concentrate first on the bedroom of the allergy sufferer and after that on other rooms in which he or she spends most of their time: improve ventilation, reduce clutter and soft toys, and strongly consider investing in good quality anti-mite barrier covers on all bedding. The rest of the house can be changed gradually, perhaps when you re-decorate a room. You should also, initially, aim to reduce humidity throughout the house by keeping the bathroom and kitchen windows open during or after use.

The Ideal Bedroom

The bedroom should be a sanctuary, a place where you can relax away from the stresses of everyday life. For many people, however, rather than feeling relaxed after a night's sleep, they wake tired, suffering with such symptoms as a blocked nose, tight chest, itchy skin or red, sore eyes.

The heat and moisture produced as you sleep, as well as the plentiful supply of skin flakes that you shed, turn your bed into the ideal breeding ground for dust mites. Every time you move, mite droppings are stirred up and breathed in, and if you are sensitive to their allergen, your allergic symptoms may worsen overnight. Similarly, contact with mite allergen in your bed may exacerbate the rash and itchiness associated with eczema.

Yet the situation is not hopeless, as you can see from the points here (see right) highlighting improvements that can be made to eliminate the dust mite from your bedroom. But as a first step, ask your doctor to test you for mite sensitivity – only if the result is positive is it worth trying to reduce the amount of dust-mite allergen in your home. Mite sensitivity, however, may not be the only cause of your allergy, so even if you take these measures, your symptoms may not completely improve.

You may not have to carry out all the recommended changes. Just one or two – especially using mite barrier covers on your mattress and bedding (see pp. 82–3) – may be enough. But you will have to persevere for several months before you can assess if there has been any real improvement.

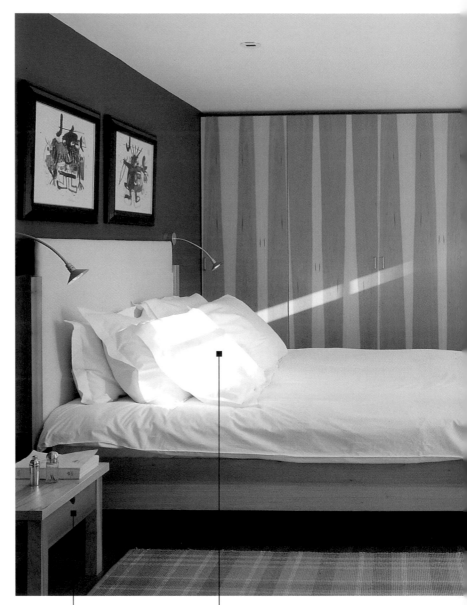

Furniture
● Keep furniture in the bedroom to a minimum, since it is all a potential dust trap.
● Choose furniture with clean, smooth lines and a minimum of detailing. This makes cleaning easier and more efficient.
● Make sure that the doors and drawers of furniture used for storing clothing and bedding close tightly, otherwise dust will work its way inside and encourage mites.
● Choose furniture that can be readily moved, in order to allow you to clean behind or underneath it.

Bedding
● Put anti-mite barrier covers on the mattress, duvet, and pillows. You must cover all the bedding to make a difference.
● Use an electric blanket, if you have one, to keep your bed dry, so helping to make it less hospitable to mites and mould.
● Replace blankets with a duvet, which can be covered with an anti-mite barrier cover. Wool or fleece underblankets should go inside the anti-mite mattress cover, but avoid using them if possible as they are difficult to wash and dry.

Walls and ornaments
● Opt for plain, simple walls, without picture rails, dado rails, or mouldings, to avoid dust collecting.
● Select wipable paint or wallpaper – any textured finishes retain dust.

● Reduce clutter on walls and ledges to a minimum to make cleaning more efficient.
● Display ornaments on shelves behind glass doors, or be prepared to damp-dust them on a weekly basis.

Window dressings
● Install roller blinds or shades, as these collect less dust than curtains or venetian blinds. Vertical venetian blinds are preferable to horizontal types.
● Use curtains that are made of cotton or muslin if you don't want blinds. Curtains made of these materials can usually be washed at high temperatures.

Windows
● Reduce humidity by leaving windows open in the morning after getting up, and preferably at night, too.
● Keep windows shut in the early morning and in the early evening if you have a pollen allergy – this is when pollen counts tend to be at their highest. Open them at other times, or if security is a problem install air conditioning or mechanical ventilation.
● Pull back the curtains on bright, sunny days – hot kills mites.

Heating
● Keep background heat on in guest or spare bedrooms to prevent condensation forming on windows or outside walls.
● Consider installing a hygrometer (humidity meter). This should ideally be kept below about 50 percent relative humidity if mites are to be discouraged.
● Consider using a vent covering to trap dust, while allowing air to pass through, if you have a forced-air heating system.

Flooring
● Replace carpets with a hard-surface flooring material, such as vinyl, linoleum, or wood, which will not harbour dust mites. Hard-surface flooring is also easier to keep clean than fitted carpets or carpet tiles.
● Use machine-washable cotton rugs in preference to woollen rugs.
● Seal the cracks between the boards of a wooden floor to prevent dust blowing up from the space beneath.
● Choose a carpet with a tightly woven short pile if you must have a carpet. Research suggests the static charge of nylon carpets helps prevent allergens from becoming airborne. Or consider buying an anti-allergy carpet (see p. 62).

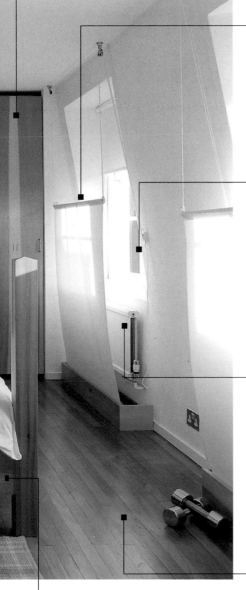

Bed
● Avoid padded headboards, especially the buttoned types, which are excellent dust traps.
● Avoid elaborate rails or fabric hangings (found on four-poster or canopy beds), which trap dust.
● Choose a raised bed to make cleaning underneath quick and easy.
● Cover your mattress completely in a dust-proof barrier cover.
● Choose a slatted base to encourage the free movement of air around the bed.

CHANGES TO MAKE

Desirable
● Cover the mattress, pillow, and duvet with anti-mite barrier covers.
● Make sure that the room is well ventilated.
● Keep pets out of the room.
● Replace carpet with hard-surface flooring.

Optional
● Replace drapes with blinds.
● Replace your old mattress, pillows, and duvet before putting on barrier covers.
● Remove soft furnishings, or at least minimize them.

CLEANING TIMETABLE

Daily
● Vacuum the floor, rugs, or carpet.
● Wipe furniture surfaces with a damp (not wet) cloth.
● Wear a dust mask if you are an allergy sufferer when making beds, cleaning, or dusting.

Weekly
● Wash bed linen using a high-temperature cycle. Non-biological washing powders may be necessary for people with eczema (see p. 21).
● Wipe barrier covers with a damp (not wet) cloth.
● Vacuum under bed to remove any mites or mite allergen.
● Clean the dust from the top of tall furniture.
● Vacuum or wipe skirting (base) boards and picture rails.

Every 3–6 months
● Wash curtains at 56°C/133°F or above.
● Wash any pillows, duvets, and blankets (unless using anti-mite covers). Make sure that bedding is thoroughly dry to prevent mould growth.

BEDDING AND BEDS

The main changes you need to make to a bedroom involve introducing physical barriers to prevent you coming into contact with mite allergen that may be present, and eliminating any mite or dust-harbouring features.

Types of bed

Beds with slatted wooden or metal bases provide better circulation of air around the mattress than divan beds. Make sure that clothes or bedding stored in divan drawers are stored in breathable plastic bags to prevent mites and dust dropping from the bed onto the clothes. Try to avoid four-poster and canopied beds, or at least replace any heavy drapes surrounding them with lightweight muslin or cotton ones, which can be washed at high temperatures to kill the mites, and damp-dust or vacuum the rails weekly. Avoid padded headboards in which mites readily breed.

Anti-mite barrier covers

Barrier covers are a proven method of avoiding exposure to mite allergen. One cover fits beneath the bottom sheet, enclosing the entire mattress, while others fit between the pillows and pillow cases and between the duvet and its cover. All bedding needs to be covered – it is simply not worth covering the mattress alone. Ideally, fit barrier covers on a new mattress and bedding before use, so that you prevent infestation right from the start.

Barrier covers prevent you coming into contact with the mite allergen contained within the fabric of your mattress and bedding. Some mites will survive on top of the cover, living on the skin scales you continually shed,

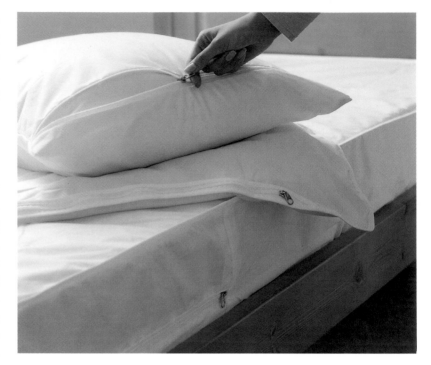

but these will be few in number and can be removed weekly by changing the sheets. This is also when you should wipe the surface of the barrier cover with a damp (not wet) cloth to remove any mites and shed skin. Wash the barrier covers about twice as year, or as advised by the manufacturer.

Old-fashioned covers are made of plastic. Although they are an effective barrier against mites and mite allergen, they do not allow water to pass through, so that you wake in the morning damp from the sweat you produced while asleep.

In contrast, modern covers are made out of a soft, microporous material that allows both water and air to pass through – although brands differ in how well they do this. Concerning durability, covers with a manufacturer's guarantee of at least 10 years are better value for money than the less expensive types that will need replacing more often.

Anti-mite barrier covers are a proven way of avoiding exposure to mite allergen, but brands vary in durability and comfort. Good ones have excellent moisture and air permeability while completely excluding mites and mite allergen.

Also available are cotton bedding covers impregnated with acaricides – chemicals that kill mites. However, little is known about the long-term effects of the chemicals on humans, and the covers do not provide a barrier to the mite allergen.

Protecting your mattress

Within three months, under the right conditions of warmth and humidity, a new mattress will be almost as infested as one that has been in use for years. One estimate has suggested that up to 2 million mites could live in a double-bed mattress. Most mites live in the uppermost layers of the mattress and some people vacuum their mattresses in the mistaken belief that they are ridding themselves of the dust mite. In fact, these tiny creatures cling to the mattress fabric and, at best, you will remove only a tiny proportion of the live mites by vacuuming.

A more effective treatment is to use a mite-killing chemical (acaricide) on the mattress and bedding. However, acaricides don't penetrate far enough to kill mites deep inside the mattress and so are not as effective as when used on carpeting. Furthermore, they need to be applied at least every three months.

Liquid nitrogen, which freezes the mites, dry steam cleaning, and heat treatment are other approaches (see pp. 70–1). All of these are unnecessary, however, if you use anti-mite barrier covers (see opposite).

Pillows and bedding

Within 12 months from new, a pillow will have increased in weight by 10 percent due to the presence of mites, mite droppings, and skin scales. In the past it was recommended that feather or down pillows and duvets should be replaced with synthetic bedding termed "non-allergenic" or "hypo-allergenic". However, there is conflicting evidence about which type of filling is best for allergy sufferers. Whether filled with foam or feathers, pillows should always be covered with barrier covers.

Bedspreads or quilts are probably best avoided as mites will breed in them, too, unless you are prepared to wash them weekly. Alternatively, in hot, sunny climates you can hang them in the sun for a few hours a week to kill the mites.

Beds that allow air to pass underneath the mattress will help discourage dust mites and mould. If you store clothes or bedding underneath your bed, they should be put be put in breathable, plastic storage bags.

TIPS FOR BUYING BARRIER COVERS

- Make sure that the manufacturer guarantees the cover to exclude completely dust-mite allergen.
- All covers should fully encase the mattress and bedding.
- Water-permeable covers allow water vapour to pass through easily, while non-breathable types (such as polyvinyl chloride) are uncomfortable to sleep on.
- Seams should be double-stitched for durability and have a good-quality zip (zipper).
- Covers should be washable using a high-temperature cycle.
- Choose covers laminated rather than coated with polyurethane and polytetrafluoroethane.

Bed linen

All sheets, pillow cases, duvet covers, and any blankets should be washed weekly. This must be at a temperature of 56°C/133°F or above to kill the mites. At lower temperatures, the mites survive, although mite allergen and dead mites will be washed out. Some people get around this problem by adding mite-killing chemicals to lower-temperature washes. Of these, benzyl benzoate is the mildest and most studied, and is, therefore, probably your best choice. However, if you prefer not to have any traces of an acaricide next to your skin, you may prefer to invest in bed linen that is washable at the right temperature to kill mites, or at least rinse the bed linen extra thoroughly if using such a product. Alternatively, freezing bedclothes for a few hours – in a domestic chest freezer – will kill the mites and allow you to use a lower wash temperature.

As an alternative to covering your pillow with a separate anti-mite barrier cover, there is now a type of pillow that comes ready-made with one. And since the material is also a physical barrier to bacteria, the pillow is also hygienic. In the future, other articles of bedding, such as duvets, may be available made out of the same material.

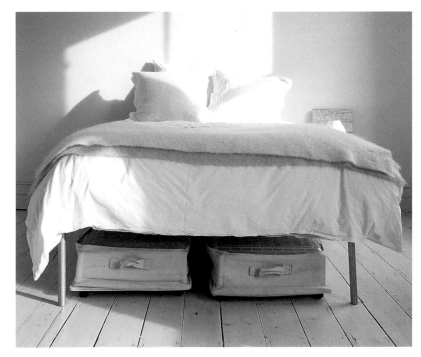

CLOTHES AND CLOTHES CARE

The invention of synthetic fibres and dyes, many based on petrochemicals, has revolutionized clothes manu-facturing. The choice of fashionable, good-quality, affordable clothing that is available today is a part of modern life we largely take for granted.

Fabric choices

There are three categories of fabrics available: natural; synthetic; and natural/synthetic mixtures. Each may repre-sent a problem to an allergy sufferer.

Natural fabrics Simply because a fabric is "natural" does not necessarily mean that it is "safe" for people with skin allergies. Wool is one example of a natural fabric that can cause intense irritation to some people. The reason for this appears to be the irritating effect of the wool fibres. Many of us, whether we have allergies or not, are familiar with the itchy feeling a woollen garment often has when worn next to the skin, an effect likely to be worse in people who already have eczema or dermatitis.

There is a popular misconception that it is the lanolin present in wool that produces the itchiness, but this is unlikely, since allergy to lanolin is rare in the general population. Nor is it particularly high among people who have skin allergies – some studies suggest that only about 1 percent of people with dermatitis are sensitive to lanolin allergens. This figure is even further decreased by the very refined,

high-grade lanolin that is used in many skin-care products and preparations made for people with dry-skin conditions. Therefore, even if you suffer with true wool sensitivity due to lanolin allergens, skin-care products containing high-grade lanolin may be used safely. Ask your pharmacist for advice on suitable products.

Natural fabrics that are not usually associated with allergic reactions and should, therefore, not cause problems are cotton, silk, and leather. Most people suffering with eczema find that cotton clothing and bedding are far more comfortable than those made from wool or synthetic fibres. This is probably because cotton causes less

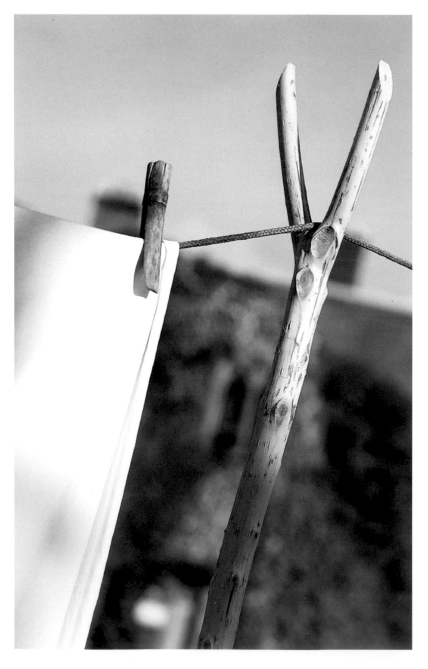

Washing should be dried outside or in a tumble drier vented to the outside. Drying washing inside over a clothes horse or radiator means that the excess moisture will go into the interior air and increase relative humidity.

sweating and skin irritation. There are specialist suppliers of unbleached, untreated cotton clothing and bedding.

Synthetics and natural/synthetic mixtures One of the commonest of the synthetic fabrics is polyester, which is also found as a component of some plastics and adhesives. Some clothes and bedding are made solely from polyester, but polyester fibres can also be combined with cotton to make what is known as polycotton. This material is frequently used for clothing, bed linen, carpeting, and as the stuffing in duvets and quilts.

Individuals can differ greatly in their tolerance of synthetics and natural/synthetic mixtures. Some people, for example, find that the types of dye used with polyester fibres irritate their skin, while polycotton and cotton products labelled "easy-care", "crease-resistant", or "non-iron" have been treated with formaldehyde (see pp. 68–71), a chemical that can cause a skin irritation in a few individuals.

Finishings and fasteners Even if you have done your homework, and have managed to avoid buying any clothes or bedding made from fabrics to which you may react, something as simple as a rough seam or edge on a garment could be enough to irritate the skin of an eczema sufferer and set up a reaction. Likewise, any exposed metal poppers, buttons, or zippers on clothes and bedding could be the trigger. Popper fasteners are popular on baby clothes, but these should be attached to the garment in such a way that they do not come into contact with the infant's skin.

Washing and drying clothes

Coloured cotton clothing or bedding should be washed before it is used for the first time in order to remove any potential irritants, such as loose dye particles. There are many washing products suitable for people with sensitive skin (see pp. 76–7).

Ideally, clothes should not be dried anywhere inside the home. This greatly increases the interior humidity and will encourage dust mite numbers and the growth of moulds. If you have no option other than to dry clothes inside the house, then choose a room that has few soft furnishings and make sure that you keep the window open and the door to the rest of the house firmly closed. Preferably, dry clothes outside or in a tumble drier, which should be vented to the outside.

Some people find that the fragrances given off by the conditioners used in tumble dryers an irritant.

Stain remover Common brands of stain remover may contain 1,1,1-trichlorethane, a solvent found in many different products, including some correcting fluids. This strong-smelling solvent evaporates rapidly and may cause sneezing or a tightening of the chest in people with respiratory allergies.

Storing clothes and footwear

Don't leave clothes lying around the bedroom to collect dust, and do not put clothes or shoes away in closets while they are damp. Placing garments on wire racks, rather than shelves, encourages air circulation and discourages mites and mould.

Fabric enclosures for clothes should be well-aired and you may need to wash them monthly, depending on how dusty the room is. Keep the doors of fitted closets closed, and avoid open hanging rails or shelves. Unused clothes should be dry and placed in breathable plastic storage bags, especially if they are to be placed in divan drawers or under beds.

The Ideal Children's Room

Parents usually put a lot of effort into decorating their children's rooms to make them interesting and stimulating. But when there is an allergic child to consider, it is also necessary to create the type of environment that will minimize symptoms.

Many of the measures dealt with here are targeted at reducing the level of dust-mite allergen, which is a common factor in allergic asthma. But before undertaking any changes you should first consult your doctor and establish that your child is, in fact, sensitive to mite allergen.

Mite-allergen control measures should be carried out in all the rooms that are used frequently by allergic children, especially their bedrooms. You should apply the measures on all the beds or bedding in the room, even if other children sharing the room do not have any symptoms of allergy. If your child's allergy is severe, you may have to consider finding a new home for any pets, especially cats. At the very least, all pets should be excluded from children's rooms or their main play areas, and kept outside as much as possible.

Couples with family histories of allergy, or who suffer from allergies themselves, may want to consider making their home into a low-allergen environment before starting a family. Research has shown that children who are born into families with a history of allergies are more likely to develop allergies, and that the level of allergen exposure during infancy is important in sensitizing a child and in the development of allergic disease.

Windows
● Air the room by opening the window in the morning, and turn back the bedclothes. Keeping the window slightly open at night helps to air the room, thus reducing humidity and discouraging mould growth and mites.
● Keep windows shut in the early morning and early evening during the pollen season if your child has a pollen allergy.
● Consider installing a single-room ventilation unit (see p. 57) if it is difficult to air the room naturally.
● Use roller blinds or shades in preference to curtains or drapes.

Furniture and furnishings
● Keep furniture to an absolute minimum to prevent a build-up of dust. Remove soft-upholstered furniture from the bedroom and replace it with furniture made from plastic or wood – materials that dust mites cannot colonize.
● Cover all cushions and pillows with barrier covers and wash ordinary covers regularly using a method that kills house-dust mites (see pp. 70–1).

Ornaments and books
● Keep shelves, windowsills, and worktops or counters clear and dust free by vacuuming or damp dusting regularly. Less clutter means less dust and easier cleaning.
● Store books and ornaments behind glass doors to prevent dust collecting on them.
● Minimize posters and other wall decorations, such as pictures and pennants, which will all collect dust.

Toys
● Keep soft toys and comfort blankets to a minimum – they can hold concentrations of dust mites sufficient to contribute to a child's asthma or eczema.
● Destroy mites by freezing soft toys or comfort blankets in a freezer for at least 3–4 hours.
● Don't let children play with modelling clay or chalk if there are any signs of it irritating their skin.
● Tidy toys away in cabinets or in toy chests at the end of every day to help keep them free from dust.
● Discard unwanted or broken toys to keep clutter to a minimum.

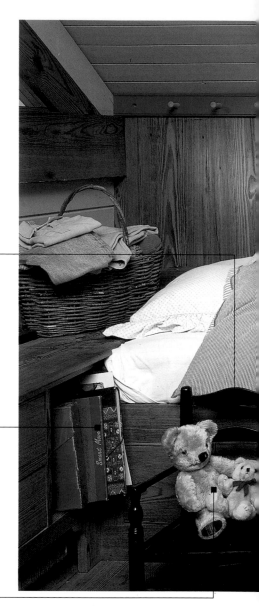

Flooring
● Replace carpets with a hard-surface flooring material, such as linoleum or wood.
● Vacuum daily, even if a hard-surface flooring material is present.
● Use washable cotton rugs instead of carpeting.

Walls
● Use quick-drying, water-based paint or low-VOC paint (*see pp. 66–9*).
● Keep children out of the room while painting and until the paint has dried. Ventilate the room until all fumes have gone.

Clothing
● Wash clothes in non-biological products or those made for sensitive skin.
● Use cotton mittens to prevent children scratching at their eczema while they are asleep.

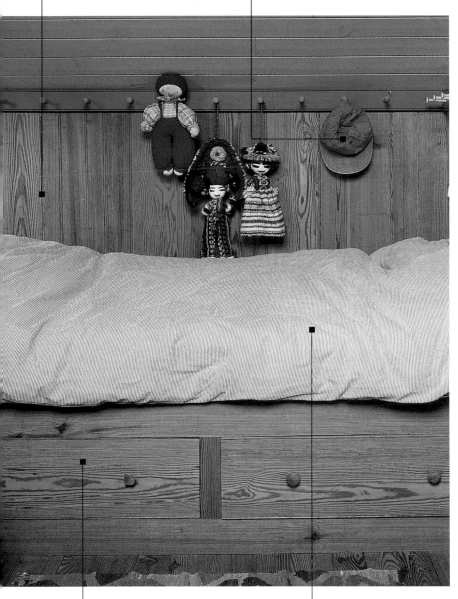

Beds
● Enclose all mattresses in barrier covers, not just the mattress of the allergic child.
● Make sure that the allergic child sleeps on the top bunk bed, if you have them.
● Keep to simple bed designs, which collect less dust, with a slatted wooden or metal base to allow air to circulate underneath the mattress.

Lampshades
● Select wipable lampshades, such as vinyl or plastic, that can easily be cleaned. Fabric shades retain dust.

Bedding
● Cover duvets and pillows with anti-mite barrier covers.
● Wash all bed linen weekly at temperatures of at least 56°C/133°F to kill mites and remove their allergen. Or add benzyl benzoate solution to washes at lower temperatures, followed by thorough rinsing.
● Use cotton sheets and blankets for children with eczema – these seem to be more comfortable than synthetic or wool fibres. Synthetic fabrics may increase sweating and wool fibres can be a skin irritant.

Desirable
● Cover all mattresses, pillows, and duvets with barrier covers.
● Replace carpets with hard flooring, such as linoleum or wood, and use washable cotton rugs for extra comfort.
● Make sure that the room is well ventilated.
● Keep soft toys to a minimum and off the beds.
● Remove soft furnishings.

Optional
● Replace curtains or drapes with roller blinds or shades.
● Store clothes outside the room.

Daily
● Vacuum hard surface floors, rugs, or carpets (*see pp. 74–5*).
● Wipe furniture surfaces with a damp (not wet) cloth.
● Try to clean when the children will be out of their room for at least a few hours, to allow any dust to settle.

Weekly
● Change bedclothes and wash them at temperatures of 56°C/133°F or above.
● Wipe barrier covers with a damp cloth every time you change the bedding.
● Freeze or wash toys.
● Vacuum under beds to remove dust that has fallen through.
● Wipe the tops of tall furniture, windowsills, or picture rails.

Every 3–6 months
● Wash curtains at temperatures of 56°C/133°F or above.
● Wash and dry pillows, duvets, blankets, and cushions, unless they have been fitted with barrier covers.
● Wash cushion and pillow covers.

ALLERGIC FACTORS

Much of the general advice given in *The Ideal Bedroom* (see pp. 80–5) applies equally to children's rooms. Remember to air rooms and beds in the morning unless you are pollen-sensitive, when you should keep windows shut at peak pollen times. Try to make beds, vacuum, and dust when any allergic children are out of their rooms. Avoid cleaning in the evenings before bed time as disturbed dust will take hours to settle out of the air.

Anti-mite barrier covers

Cover mattresses, duvets, and pillows in anti-mite barrier covers (see pp. 82–3). All beds in the room should be treated in this way – even those of non-allergic children, since their bedding will also harbour dust mites and their allergen.

Bed linen should be changed weekly and washed at a high temperature (56°C/133°F or above) to kill the dust mite and remove the allergen. Other bedclothes, such as bedspreads, must also be washed weekly at high temperatures.

In hot, sunny climates an alternative to washing thicker bedclothes, such as quilts or bedspreads, on a weekly basis is to hang them in strong sunlight for several hours each week. The sunlight should kill most of the mites, and so reduce the amount of allergen produced. The remaining allergen will have to be washed out, possibly at only 3-monthly intervals.

The duvets and pillows themselves do not need regular washing if they have been covered with barrier covers. However, you will have to wipe the cover with a damp (but not wet) cloth to remove dust mites

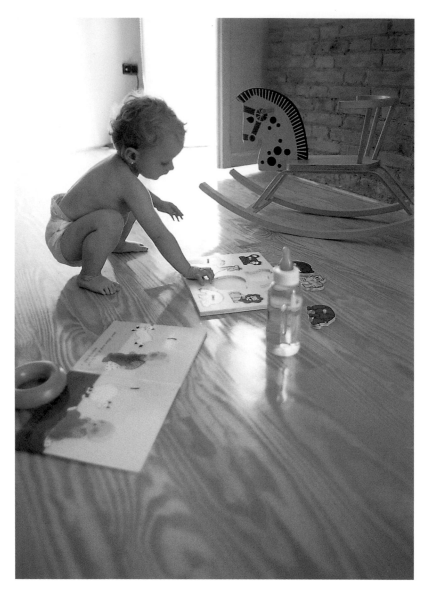

every time you change the bedding. Modern barrier covers are water permeable, so if a child wets the bed you will need to strip off all the bedding and wash it. Thorough drying of bedclothes is important, especially of thicker items such as quilts, to eliminate any risk of dampness and, therefore, mould growth.

Bunk and divan beds

If bunk beds are used, the allergic child should sleep on the top bed, as dust

If your baby suffers from diaper rash (diaper dermatitis), caused by the ammonia in urine, cover the affected area with a water-repellent barrier cream and leave the diaper off as much as possible until the rash has healed.

mites and allergen will drift down from the top bunk on to the child below. Divan beds inhibit the circulation of air beneath the mattress, and so any clothes or toys stored in drawers beneath the bed should be in breathable plastic storage bags to prevent mite colonization.

Cots (cribs)

Although the same cot (crib) can be used for different babies over the years, each infant should have his or her own new mattress. Replace any mattress, however, if any signs of mould (black stains) develop. This will happen if it is not thoroughly dried out after becoming wet.

Cot (crib) mattresses are usually made of foam, though some people prefer a natural cotton stuffing. A foam mattress is usually partly covered with a vinyl plastic to protect it against soiling, while the section where the baby lays its head is left uncovered for safety reasons. Barrier covers for cot (crib) mattresses are available from specialist suppliers. Do not use home-made plastic covers – these are unsafe and may cause suffocation.

When allergic children move from a cot (crib) to their first "proper" bed they should start off with a new mattress, duvet, and pillow, which should all be protected with barrier covers to keep them mite-free right from the beginning. There is, however, a new heat-treatment procedure that can be used to clean old mattresses and bedding to kill dust mites and denature their droppings, so that they are no longer allergenic (see p. 71).

Soft toys

Piles of soft toys in a bedroom are a health hazard for any child with a mite allergy. Just like soft furnishings and carpets, cuddly toys create an ideal breeding environment for mites. Soft toys should be tidied away in a closet or chest at night rather than kept on the bed or cot (crib). You may, however, need to make an exception for a child's favourite toy or blanket.

Keep soft toys in the bedroom to a minimum and, ideally, wash them weekly at water temperatures of 56°C/133°F or above. Toys can be washed at lower temperatures if a solution of mite-killing benzyl benzoate is used (see p. 76) – but

since favourite toys are likely to be sucked and in constant contact with the child, some parents may not be happy with this option. Alternatively, you can place soft toys inside a plastic bag and leave them in your refrigerator's freezer compartment for 3–4 hours. This will kill all the mites, but you will still have to wash their droppings away.

If you wash or freeze toys weekly right from new, dust mites will never have the opportunity to establish themselves in any great numbers, especially if you use barrier covers on all bedding so that there are no reservoirs of dust mite in the room to recolonize the clean toys.

Apply this regime, more or less strictly, to soft toys that are kept in other rooms, depending on how often the child plays with them. Carrying out this routine does require time and effort, and it may be easier to keep only a few soft toys, which you can then rotate through the anti-mite regime.

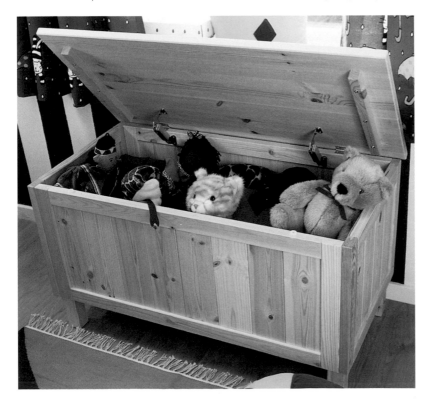

Placing soft toys in a chest when not in use helps to keep them free of dust and makes the room easier to clean. This chest is made of solid wood and does not have the problems associated with board products (see p. 71).

The Ideal Living Room

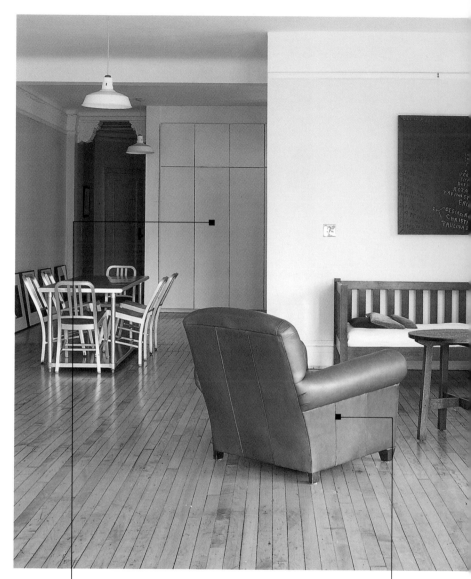

The living or family room is normally where the whole family can relax in comfort. Depending on personal taste, it may be carpeted or have a hard-surface floor, perhaps covered with rugs. Furniture will probably include upholstered sofas (couches) and chairs and scatter cushions or pillows. There is likely to be a television and a sound system. On the walls, there will be paintings, prints, or photographs – perhaps even wall-hangings. Ornaments will be in display cabinets, on shelves around the room, or arranged on the mantlepiece. Some older homes may still have their original open fires. Although this sounds very pleasant, there are factors that could make life less than comfortable for allergy sufferers.

Chief among these are the type of flooring and the presence of soft furnishings, including upholstered sofas or couches and curtains. Very important, too, is whether or not a pet is allowed access to the room, the ease with which the arrangement of the room permits regular cleaning, and the type of materials used in the construction of cabinets or shelves.

You must first identify the allergy sufferer's specific needs before you can undertake effective controls. If, for example, sensitivity to mite allergen is a crucial element in a person's symptoms, then mite control will be the key to adapting the room. However, people with animal allergies need to reconsider the place of any animals in the home, while sufferers from mould allergies may be helped by preventing mould growth due to condensation.

Furniture
● Choose furniture that fits to the ceiling.
● Avoid open shelves. Bookshelves should have glass doors.
● Air new board-based furniture (see p. 71) to reduce levels of formaldehyde gas.

Sound and TV equipment
● Store electric equipment in cabinets.
● Choose a vacuum cleaner that can be used for cleaning electrical equipment.
● Check that cockroaches cannot gain access to the insides of electric equipment, where they can live undetected, producing a build-up of allergen.

Sofas (couches) and armchairs
● Buy sofas and chairs covered in material that dust mites cannot colonize, such as leather or vinyl.
● Keep your fabric-upholstered furniture to a minimum. Vacuuming this type of furniture may remove some mite allergen but it will have little effect on the live mites, and so the effort is difficult to justify.
● Use cotton throws over any fabric-upholstered furniture you keep. Wash the throws weekly to monthly to remove mites and allergen. Alternatively, you may want to try adapting anti-mite barrier covers for your sofa or couch from those sold specifically for bedding (see pp. 82–3).

Walls and lighting
● Keep mouldings and skirting (base) boards simple to avoid dust traps. For the same reason, choose plain, non-textured wallpaper or smooth paint finishes.
● Avoid pendant light fixtures, such as chandeliers, or fabric lampshades, unless you are prepared to clean and dust them regularly. Choose table lamps that are easy to wipe free of dust, or install easy-to-clean inset lighting, such as halogen lamps.

Ornaments and books
● Keep ornaments and knick-knacks to a minimum – they collect less dust and make thorough cleaning difficult.
● Place ornaments behind glass in a display cabinet, if possible.

Windows
● Keep the room well ventilated by leaving trickle ventilators open (if you have modern windows) or simply by opening windows (see pp. 52–9).
● Hang lightweight, washable curtains in preference to heavy or lined drapes. Curtains should be washable at temperatures of 56°C/133°F, or above, or install easy-to-clean roller blinds or shades.
● Consider installing double (secondary) glazing in a new home or when replacing windows. This will provide better insulation against heat loss as well as prevent condensation, which may, in turn, lead to the growth of mould.

Cushions (pillows)
● Cover cushions in material that is washable at temperatures of 56°C/133°F, or above, or fit cushions with anti-mite barrier cover.
● Dry washed cushions thoroughly – preferably in a tumble dryer – to prevent the possibility of mould growing inside the damp stuffing.

Heating
● Consider installing underfloor heating, or radiant heating in the form of panels on the walls or within the skirting (base) boards (see pp. 60–1), when building a new home or undertaking major redecoration.
● Don't install forced-air central heating or rely on fan or convector heaters if dust is a major problem in the room. Conventional radiators may be better in this situation, but make sure that you vacuum the dust that inevitably collects behind them.

Fireplaces
● Choose a simply designed electric fire that has few hard-to-clean features where dust can accumulate.
● Maintain open fires regularly to prevent combustion by-products venting back into the room. Smokeless fuel is preferable to coal, which may produce high levels of sulphur dioxide.

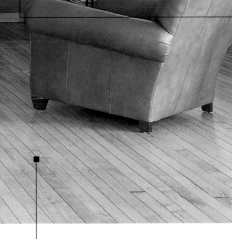

Flooring
● Install hard-surface flooring (such as solid wood, laminated wood, or linoleum) in preference to wall-to-wall carpeting or carpet tiles, which rapidly become a dust-mite reservoir. For comfort, use cotton rugs that can be washed at water temperatures of 56°C/133°F, or above.
● Seal cracks and gaps in wooden floors to make them easy to clean. This also prevents dust blowing up from the spaces beneath the floor.
● If you have carpet, vacuum with a HEPA vacuum cleaner (see pp. 74–5) or install an anti-allergy carpet (see p. 62).

CHANGES TO MAKE

Desirable
● Install a hard-surface flooring material, such as wood, when the time comes to replace your carpet.
● Replace fabric-covered soft furnishings with leather or vinyl equivalents.
● Replace heavy, lined drapes with lightweight, washable curtain material, or easy-to-clean roller blinds or shades.

Optional
● Avoid placing ornaments on open shelving. They will attract dust and be difficult to keep clean.
● Fit glass doors to existing open bookshelves to minimize the build-up of dust.
● Replace curtains with blinds or shades.

CLEANING TIMETABLE

Daily
● Vacuum hard-surface flooring or wipe it with a damp cloth.
● If you have a fitted carpet, it is best to vacuum all of it – not just the heavily used parts.
● Damp-dust furniture surfaces.

Weekly
● Damp-dust out-of-the-way surfaces, such as the tops of cabinets, pictures and dado rails, and ornaments on open diplay. Wipe down leather chairs.
● Polish furniture (as required), avoiding scented products.

Every 3–6 months
● Consider cleaning fabric furnishings and carpets to kill dust mites. Vacuum thoroughly afterwards to remove dead mites and mite allergen.
● Wash lightweight curtains or wipe down blinds or shades.

ALLERGIC FACTORS

The most crucial factors determining the levels of mite allergens in the living room are the type of flooring material used and the style of furniture and curtaining. As well as affecting the level of mite allergen, furniture can also be a source of formaldehyde, which is an irritant gas that provokes symptoms, such as sneezing or coughing, in allergic individuals who are hyperresponsive to this substance. Modern furniture, including cabinets, tables, and shelving, is often made from board material, such as medium-density fibreboard, and is an important source of formaldehyde in the home (see p. 69). The underlay of foam-backed carpets also contains formaldehyde.

Hard-surface floors

The best type of flooring for a low-allergen living room is a hard surface one, such as wood or linoleum. However, if the allergy sufferer does not use the room regularly, carpeting may be acceptable – although in these circumstances an anti-allergy carpet may be worth considering (see p. 62). For extra comfort on a hard surface floor, you can use machine-washable cotton rugs rather than wool rugs, which require more specialized cleaning. Make sure that you fix rugs securely to any type of hard surface floor to prevent them slipping when stepped on.

When cleaning wood or linoleum floors, remember that heavily scented home-care products, such as many detergents and polishes, can in themselves trigger an irritant reaction in sensitive individuals. If this is a problem, there are non-scented products available from which to choose.

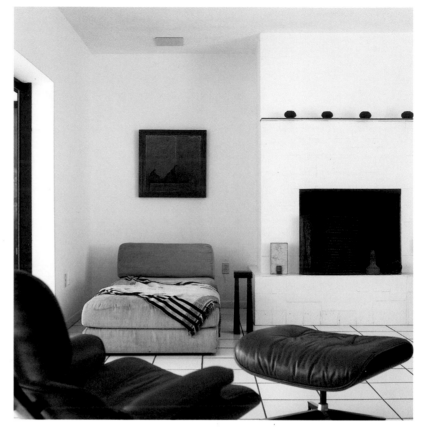

Only sealed wooden floors should be washed – all gaps between the boards have to be filled (this will prevent dust blowing up from below) and the surface of the wood treated with an appropriate product to prevent water penetration. Even so, wring out mops or sponges until they are just damp to avoid excessively wetting the wood. Repair any worn or poorly sealed areas of flooring, as water penetrating the boards may cause the wood to warp.

Carpets

For allergy sufferers, carpeting can be important as a reservoir for dust mites and mould. If your allergic symptoms are pronounced in the presence of these agents, consider removing carpets from rooms you regularly use. However, if your allergic

Ideal low-allergen features in a living room include hard surface flooring and leather- or vinyl-upholstered furniture, both of which do not harbour dust mites and are easily cleaned. Any fabric throws should be machine washable.

reaction is only mild, undertaking a regime of regular carpet vacuuming and periodic cleaning may be enough to keep symptoms under control.

Wet washing Domestic carpet washing machines may remove mites and allergen along with dirt, but may ultimately result in more mites as the water left at the base of the carpet pile or in the carpet underlay greatly increases humidity, thus encouraging mite numbers and the growth of mould. However, professional carpet washing is usually very efficient at removing the water used and the carpet should dry out quickly, provided there is good ventilation.

Dry cleaning Solvents are sprayed directly on to the carpet or rug to loosen the dirt, which is then removed using a second solution containing ionizers. Optical brighteners and other chemicals such as deodorizers may be added. Dry cleaning kills mites but some people with allergies may find the process has an irritant effect on their symptoms. It may be necessary to stay away during professional cleaning and to air the house well afterwards.

Dry powder solvents are an alternative to wet solvents. These are sprinkled on to lightly dampened carpets and left for a short time to absorb the dirt before being vacuumed off. It can be difficult, even using a powerful vacuum cleaner, to remove all the powder, which may then be left behind to irritate the skin or airways of sensitive individuals.

Anti-mite chemicals These aim to kill mites or neutralize mite allergen (so it no longer causes an allergic reaction) but used alone do not reduce allergic symptoms (see p. 70).

Steam treatment Several steam methods kill dust mites, but not all neutralize mite allergen. One newly developed method boils ordinary tapwater (piped water) under pressure to produce very hot steam, which them penetrates deep into the pile to kill mites. There is evidence to show this method denatures mite allergen. As the steam contains very little

water, it is sometimes described as "dry" steam. Afterward, the dead mites and allergen are vacuumed away. Steam treatment may be used to treat fabric upholstery and curtains as well, but should be tested on a small area first to make sure the carpet or fabric is not affected by the process.

Soft furnishings

Fabric-covered furnishings provide the perfect environment for mites and should be replaced with leather or vinyl coverings, which can be wiped down with a damp cloth weekly to remove dust and mites. Being realistic, it is likely that you will have some fabric-covered furnishings, even if only a few scatter cushions (pillows). Ready-made anti-mite barrier covers are available for pillows and bedding (see pp. 82–3), and these can be adapted for sofas (couches) and armchairs. See pages 70–1 for other approaches to mite control, such as the use of acaricides and liquid nitrogen.

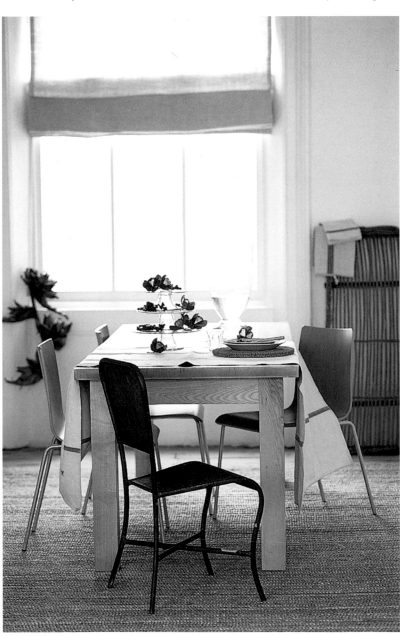

Living rooms often include an area for dining. The furniture here is unfussy and easy to keep clean. No fabric upholstery has been used, to help deter dust mites, and an easy-clean blind or shade has replaced more traditional curtains.

The Ideal Kitchen

Some kitchens are galley-sized, intended just for storing and preparing food, while others are family rooms incorporating a dining area. Some are used more or less constantly throughout the day, while others are empty apart from an hour or so in the morning over breakfast. No matter what size or type of kitchen you have, there are important factors to consider when designing a low-allergen environment. In particular, your choice of cooker (stove) or range has an impact on the level of air pollution. From an allergy point of view, cooking with electricity is far better than gas or solid fuel, which produce large amounts of combustion by-products and water vapour.

The kitchen is known as a "wet" room, due to the amount of water vapour produced by such everyday activities as cooking, boiling kettles (pans), and so on. Reducing the amount of water escaping into the home by improving ventilation (see pp. 52–7) has an important knock-on effect, reducing overall humidity levels and, thus, limiting dust mite numbers and mould growth in all rooms.

Your choice of flooring has a direct effect on dust mite numbers, with hard floor surfaces providing a less-friendly environment than carpet or carpet tiles. A hard floor is also easier to keep clean, which is an important consideration where spills and food scraps will be happily received by any lurking cockroaches (see pp. 38–9). Bear in mind that, worldwide, cockroaches are second only to the house-dust mite as a cause of allergy.

Walls
- Choose flat, smooth surfaces – they collect less dust and are easier to keep clean than textured surfaces.
- Use washable paint on the walls, and put tiles behind the range or cooker (stove) to act as an easy-clean splashback.
- Keep walls free of clutter as much as possible – pictures, decorative plates, posters, ornaments, and so on are dust and grease collectors.
- Tile areas of wall that are adjacent to worktops or counters to make the area easier to keep clean.

Windows
- Open windows or add a powered extractor (exhaust) fan to improve air exchange and minimize condensation when the kitchen is in use.
- Use roller blinds, shades, or washable curtains, not heavy drapes.

Refrigerators and freezers
- Regularly empty any water that has collected in the drip pan under the refrigerator to prevent mould growth and discourage cockroaches.
- Keep cooling coils clean and free from dust and dirt.

Kitchen furniture
- Use easy-clean furniture, such as wood, plastic, vinyl, leather, and glass.
- Sweep or vacuum under the table and chairs on a daily basis to eliminate food sources for cockroaches.
- Cover any upholstered furniture in material that can be washed at 56°C/133°F, or above – the temperature needed to kill dust mites.

Flooring
- Choose hard-surface flooring, such as linoleum, wood, or glazed tiles, in preference to carpet or carpet tiles.
- Flooring must fit neatly around the bases of cabinets for easy cleaning.
- Clean spills or dropped food immediately.

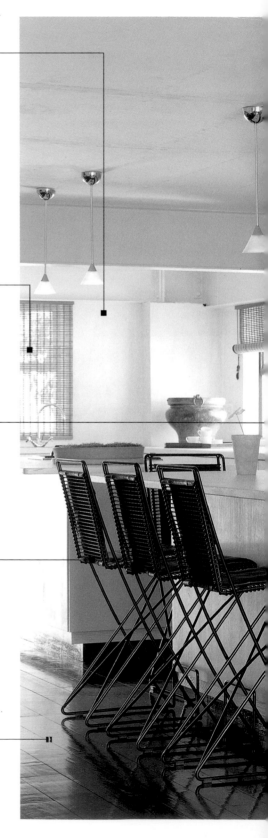

Lighting
● Avoid difficult-to-clean fluorescent strip lighting or fabric-covered lampshades and install easy-to-clean inset halogen lighting (with glass covers) or glass globes.
● Bear in mind that lighting situated above the range or cooker, or built into the cooker hood, will need more frequent cleaning.

Kitchen cabinets
● Choose stainless-steel, solid-wood, or low-emission board cabinets, or those sealed entirely with plastic laminate. Ready-made cabinets are often produced from board products that emit formaldehyde (see p. 71).
● Keep clutter and ornaments to a minimum to prevent dust collecting and make surfaces easier to clean.
● Build kitchen cabinets right up to the ceiling to avoid dust-collecting, hard-to-clean tops.

Cookers or ranges and hoods
● Buy an electric cooker (stove) or range rather than a gas or solid-fuel type.
● Minimize condensation by keeping lids on pans and don't over-boil.
● Bear in mind that a ducted hood removes excess moisture to the outside, while a recirculating hood does not.
● Change or clean filters as recommended by the manufacturer to maintain efficiency.

Kitchen sink and drainer
● Consider a water softener, which may benefit eczema sufferers living in hard-water areas. But never give children artificially softened water or mix it with milk formulas because of its high salt content.
● Replace tap (faucet) washers and secure any leaky connections. Reducing water availability will help to prevent cockroach infestation.
● Keep sink strainers clear to eliminate a food source for cockroaches.
● Place non-organic dust – silica gel or boric acid – in cracks and crevices under the sink area (and elsewhere) to control cockroaches.

Worktop or counter surfaces
● Keep food surfaces (and kitchen appliances) free of food debris to prevent mould and cockroach infestation.
● Minimize clutter and dust by putting things away in cabinets.
● Use water-resistant grouting for tiled worktops or counters.
● Make sure grouting is flush with the tile surface to prevent food building up in cracks.

CHANGES TO MAKE

Desirable
● Replace carpeting or carpet tiles with a hard floor surface.
● Install an extractor (exhaust) hood vented to the outside.
● Reduce clutter on open shelves to reduce dust.

Optional
● Replace curtains or drapes with washable blinds or shades.
● Replace soft furnishings with non-fabric materials.
● Replace a gas or solid-fuel cooker (stove) or range with electric.

CLEANING TIMETABLE

Daily
● Vacuum and mop the floor.
● Clear away food and used utensils as you work.
● Wipe up spills as they occur.
● Wipe down food-preparation surfaces with a cloth that has been dampened with disinfectant solution.
● Empty waste containers.
● Wipe the oven clean after use if it needs it.

Weekly
● Clean the refrigerator.
● Clean the drip pan of the refrigerator/freezer.
● Clean all surfaces adjacent to food-preparation areas, windowsills, and skirting (base) boards.

Every 1–3 months
● Wash cotton drapes or clean blinds or shades.
● Check cabinets for out-of-date food and remove.

Every 3–6 months
● Defrost the freezer.
● Wash down walls, ceiling, and kitchen cabinets.

KEY FEATURES

The main features of a kitchen likely to affect the frequency or severity of an allergy sufferer's symptoms are the type of cooking method used and the room's ventilation.

Hobs (cooktops), ovens, and ranges

Cooking generates significant amounts of interior air pollution by producing vapours and airborne particulate matter, such as grease. In addition, food particles that fall on to the burners are incinerated, releasing combustion by-products.

Although many people prefer to cook with gas, electric appliances are better in terms of air quality. Gas-fuelled appliances, in which the flame is open to the room's air, are a significant source of air pollution in the home. Burning gas releases water vapour as well as carbon monoxide, carbon dioxide, nitrogen dioxide, sulphur dioxide, and aldehydes.

If you cannot replace your cooker (stove), the following measures will help minimize the amount of pollution caused by burning gas:

- Appliances with electronic ignition are better than types that have constantly burning pilot lights, in terms both of fuel consumption and the emission of combustion gases. New models should be equipped with electronic ignition.
- Control the flame so that it is confined under the base of the pan.
- Follow the guidelines for interior air quality and ventilation (see pp. 52–9).
- Use an extractor (exhaust) hood vented to the outside or open a window when cooking.

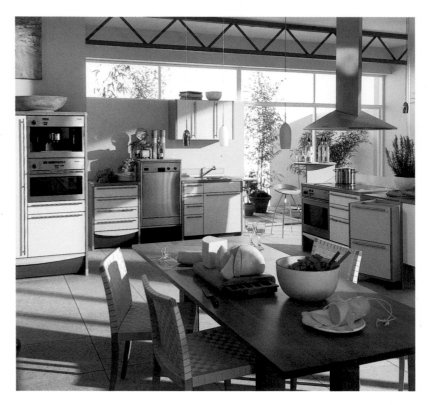

- Keep connecting doors shut while cooking to stop fumes and condensation spreading into the rest of the home

Some of the features that should be included as part of the design for a low-allergen kitchen include clutter-free surfaces, easy-to-clean furniture, hard surface flooring, a cooker (stove) or range hood, and efficient ventilation.

There are a few gas appliances – some types of range oven, for example – that have a balanced flue. This means that combustion by-products, including water vapour, are exhausted directly to the outside.

Oven cleaning

Products designed for cleaning ovens are another common source of air pollution in the kitchen, with most proprietary cleaners giving off irritating fumes. Safer methods of cleaning are available (see p. 76).

Many ovens have self-cleaning linings. These either oxidize the grease and dirt splashed on to them during cooking or burn it off. Burning grease and dirt may cause unpleasant fumes, which can irritate respiratory allergies. Some ovens use steam to loosen dirt, which you then need to wipe out.

Cooking methods

Always put lids on pans and use only as much water as is required. This reduces the amount of condensation produced as well as saving energy. A layered steamer cooks different vegetables simultaneously on a single burner, producing less condensation.

A pressure cooker cooks food rapidly by increasing air pressure and raising the water temperature. As well as saving energy, pressure cooking also conserves more food nutrients than conventional cooking. Stir-frying in a wok is another energy-efficient way to cook food. It also conserves nutrients and, because of the rapid cooking time, minimizes pollutants.

There are no allergy-based reasons for avoiding microwave ovens.

Cooker (stove) hoods

These hoods are designed to suck up steam, grease, and odours, and must be installed at the height recommended by the manufacturer for maximum effectiveness. Most models have a variable speed control. Ask to hear the hood working before buying it. One consumer study found that operating noise was the main reason why people did not use their hoods. Those with remote fans are quieter.

Ducted hoods   Some cooker (stove) hoods are ducted to the outside, thus ensuring that all combustion by-products and excess condensation are removed from the home. Air is sucked up from above the hob (cooktop) and passed through a grease filter before being expelled to the outside. The filter, which can be made of foam, metal, or special paper, must either be regularly washed or replaced, and the ductwork to the outside should be as short and straight as possible.

It is important to have an opening window or some other source of clean air, such as a window ventilator, to replace the air removed by a ducted hood. If not, the hood will suck air from the rest of the house along the path of least resistance. This may

be down the open flue of a boiler or water heater in or near the kitchen, and the resulting replacement air would then be many times more polluted than that being exhausted.

Unlike balanced-flue appliances (*see p. 61*), an open flue uses air from the room for combustion, and then expels combustion by-products up a chimney or flue. Whenever an open-flued appliance is installed in a house with an extractor (exhaust) such as a hood, a test should be carried out to ensure that combustion by-products cannot be sucked back in. If you install a hood after gas appliances have been fitted, make sure this test is performed.

Recirculating hoods   There is no danger of air being sucked down an open flue by extractor (exhaust) hoods that recirculate air back into the kitchen via a filter. However, although these models do remove grease and odours, they do not remove excess moisture and thus do not reduce humidity. If you cannot replace the hood with a ducted type, make sure that there is good ventilation during cooking by opening a window or outside door; but keep the door to the rest of the home shut to prevent moisture escaping into other rooms. If you choose a new cooker (stove) or range hood, take the following into consideration:

- Noise level when switched on
- Variability of speed control
- Ease of cleaning/replacing filters and cleaning the hood itself
- Ducted models are preferable to recirculating types

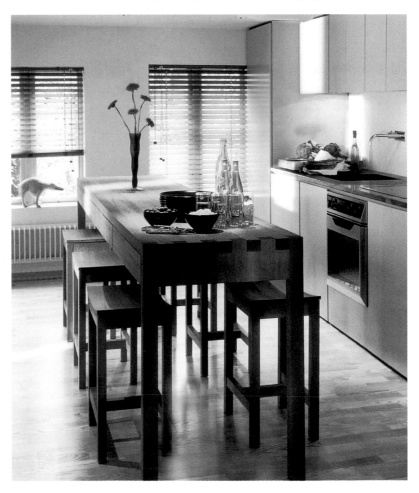

This low-allergen kitchen has cabinets built up to the ceiling to prevent dust collecting on top, wipable blinds (shades), solid wood furniture that can be wiped free of dust, and a laminated floor to deny mites a home.

Kitchen furniture

Kitchen cabinets are often made from board products, such as chipboard (particle board), which give off high concentrations of formaldehyde vapour when new (*see p. 71*). Choose cabinets made from laminated board, a solid softwood, or from stainless steel. Ceramic or quarry tiles, granite, marble, or solid wood can all be used for worktops (counters).

Refrigerators and freezers

Check inside and under your refrigerator and freezer, especially the door seals, and clean if necessary. The drip pan should be easily accessible for emptying and cleaning. You need to do this weekly to stop bacteria and mould from growing. Emptying the drip pan also removes a water source for cockroaches. Keeping cooling coils clean, so that they don't become coated with dust, saves energy as well as helping to improve air quality.

Try to buy as much natural fresh food as possible, especially vegetables and fruit. These are rich in antioxidants compared with processed foods, which contain high levels of preservatives and additives. It has been shown that there are reduced incidences of allergic disease in communities where a lot of natural fresh food is eaten.

Fly-killers

Toxic chemicals from solid block or aerosol fly killers contaminate the air and any uncovered food, while some fly sprays are respiratory irritants. Home-made flypapers can be made by boiling equal parts of sugar, corn

A streamlined kitchen design makes surfaces easy to keep clean. Note the spacious cupboards that swing open without the need for handles, while the tightly fitting cabinets prevent cockroaches creeping in.

syrup, and water together and then spreading the resulting mixture on paper strips. When the mixture has set to a sticky consistency, hang the strips up near doors and windows.

Some fresh herbs, such as basil (*Ocimum basilicum*), rosemary (*Rosmarinus*), and thyme (*Thymus*), are also said to deter flies. Instead of spraying potentially toxic chemicals into the air, why not grow pots of these aromatic herbs on the windowsill, where they would also be conveniently to hand for cooking? Dried orange peel, lemon peel, and cloves stored in open jars will also

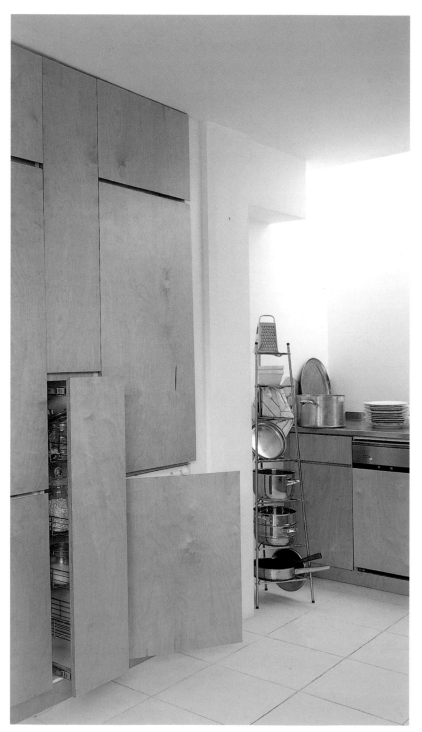

act as a fly deterrent, as do fly screens over windows or doors. If the screens face windward, they also help to trap dust.

Water softeners

Moving to a soft-water area, or installing a water softener, can improve the symptoms of eczema. Soft water, either natural or artificially softened, helps to reduce the amount of detergents, soaps, and washing powders you need to use, and the amount of scaling in pipes and kettles. However, don't give artificially softened water to children to drink and don't use it to make up formula milk for babies because it has an increased salt content.

Cleaning products

Many kitchen cleaning products, especially strongly scented ones, can irritate asthma or rhinitis conditions, while people with eczema may find that some types of washing powders and fabric conditioners irritate their skin condition (see pp. 76-7).

Animals

If any member of the family is allergic to dogs or cats it is best not to have them anywhere in the home. If total

---

PREVENTING THE GROWTH OF MOULD

- Clean all areas where moulds might grow with a bleach solution and then treat with a mould inhibitor.
- Make sure that all window frames are properly sealed and replace any rotten frames or cracked boarding.
- Remove rotting food.
- Clean work surfaces thoroughly of all crumbs and food debris.
- Wash out the bottom of the rubbish bin (trash can) regularly.
- Keep humidity as low as possible – the commonest moulds in the home

are those belonging to the *Aspergillus* spp. and the *Penicillium* spp., both of which thrive in air that is above 70 percent relative humidity.
- Check for signs of mould behind furniture, in cupboards and hidden in drawers.
- Check inside and under your freezer and refrigerator, especially the door seals, and clean them if necessary.
- Be careful not to drop food in awkward, hard-to-reach areas where mould will grow undisturbed.

---

exclusion is not possible, then confine them to the garden or at least the kitchen, which has few of the soft coverings that mites love. Bear in mind that cat dander is particularly potent at causing symptoms, compared with dog dander, because it stays airborne for longer and is much more widespread in the home.

Some dog breeds seem to cause less of an allergic reaction than others, in particular those that do not moult their coats, such as poodles and bichon frisés. Grooming your pet outside and washing it, and its bedding, twice weekly will help to reduce the amount of allergen in the home.

Some dogs are allergic to dust mite-allergen, and research suggests

about 30–40 percent of dogs suffer from mite-related eczema. This is usually treated with expensive immuno-therapy or steroid creams, but symptoms can often be relieved by covering the dog's bedding with the same type of barrier cover used for human bedding (see pp. 82–3). Some allergy product specialists supply barrier covers especially for dog bedding, but otherwise a pillow-sized barrier cover would provide the same protection, even if it is a loose fit.

In areas of cockroach infestation, pets should be fed at particular times of the day, and the food cleaned up promptly after every meal. Keep pet food in resealable containers and don't leave water out all the time.

PREVENTING COCKROACH INFESTATION

Moisture
- Reduce dampness, making improvements to ventilation if necessary (see pp. 52–9).
- Don't leave bowls of water out all the time for pets, and cover fish tanks, which can be a source of moisture for cockroaches.
- Wipe away condensation under the refrigerator every time you empty the drip pan.
- Tighten any loose pipes and repair plumbing leaks, especially around

kitchen sinks and dishwashers, to deprive the insects of water.

Food
- Dispose of waste food promptly and keep food-preparation areas clean.
- Keep food in sealed containers or in the refrigerator.
- Vacuum regularly to remove food crumbs, especially in eating areas.
- Feed your pet at regular times and clean up after every meal.
- Keep sink strainers clean and empty.

- Clear away all dirty dishes immediately after use.
- Keep kitchen appliances free of crumbs and food scraps.

Access
- Seal cracks and crevices in walls and in the woodwork around doors and windows.
- Seal any gaps around piping. Cockroaches migrate using the pipework running between properties or flats (apartments).

The Ideal Bathroom

For many people, the bathroom is where they can luxuriate, stretched full-length in a steaming bath, or stand as the shower massages the tensions away. As well as being somewhere private and relaxing, the bathroom should also be a healthy place for those with allergies. And, generally speaking, this is the case.

Most bathrooms are sparsely furnished and have easily dried, hard-surface floors, such as linoleum, vinyl, or tiles. Such a space is an inhospitable place for the dust mite, and is also somewhere that is easy to keep clean provided that you observe the general rule about minimizing clutter.

Along with the kitchen (see pp. 94–9), the bathroom is regarded as a "wet" room because of the amount of water vapour produced by such everyday activities as bathing or washing. During and after bathing or showering, keep the door firmly closed between the bathroom and the rest of the home. This will greatly reduce the amount of water vapour escaping; and if you leave a window in the bathroom open, or fit a powered extractor (exhaust) fan, most of the water vapour will escape outside.

The amount of moisture produced in a bathroom makes it an attractive proposition for cockroaches (see pp. 38–9). Worldwide, cockroaches are second only to the house-dust mite as a cause of allergies, and one of the best ways of combatting them is to deprive them of moisture. In cockroach-prone regions, this means drying sinks, baths, and shower cubicles immediately after use.

Ornaments and decorations
● Keep ornaments and pictures to a minimum to prevent dust accumulating.
● Choose succulents or other types of plant that require little watering. A dry soil surface is not likely to encourage the growth of mould.

Medicine cabinet
● Take particular care to keep all medicines out of the reach of children in a secure medicine cabinet. Bear in mind that certain medications can provoke asthma attacks. This occurs most often with medicines containing aspirin, non-steroidal anti-inflammatory tablets, and beta-blockers used for heart disease (tablets) or for glaucoma (eye-drops).
● Be aware that some people are allergic to antibiotics, such as penicillin. In severe cases, this may lead to anaphylactic shock (see pp. 22–3).

Bath
● Make sure that you thoroughly rinse away the residue of whatever you use to clean your bath and sink, especially if you have sensitive skin or eczema. Consider using a tolerated shampoo to clean the bath, especially if it is greasy from using bath oil or emollient: wipe on undiluted, scrub, and then rinse clean with the shower attachment.
● Add specially prepared bath oil to the water before bathing if you have eczema.

Toilet
● Always wear protective gloves when using the products sold for cleaning toilet bowls, and provide good ventilation. These are often powerful chemicals, some of which may irritate respiratory or skin conditions. Do not use sprays at all if they provoke respiratory symptoms.

Flooring
● Choose a hard surface flooring, such as sealed wood or cork, tiles, vinyl, or linoleum.
● Use washable cotton rugs in preference to wall-to-wall carpet or carpet tiles. Carpet will not dry easily if it becomes damp, and the moisture may encourage the rapid growth of the dust-mite population, as well as mould.

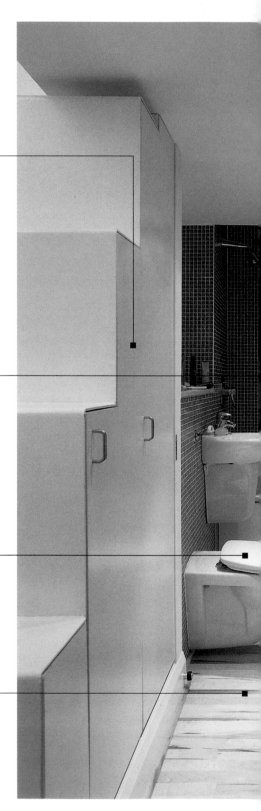

Windows

● Install frosted glass rather than blinds (shades) or curtains (drapes), for privacy. If you have a clear glass window, a roller blind (shade) is easier to keep clean of dust and mould than curtains (drapes).

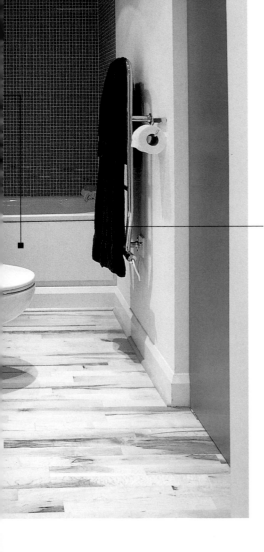

● Reduce condensation by opening a window during bathing (and leave it open afterward until all condensation has cleared), or install a powered extractor (exhaust) fan (see p. 55). Double- (secondary-) glazing also prevents condensation forming.

Walls

● Use washable and waterproof wallpaper or paint on walls and ceiling.
● Install tiling around the bath and as a splashback for the sink. Tiles are easy to clean and dry rapidly.
● Avoid ornate mouldings, skirting (base) boards, dado rails, and other features that will become dust traps.

Shower and shower curtain

● Make sure that shower curtains dry quickly after use to inhibit the growth of mould. If mould does develop, remove it by rubbing in a paste made from one-third cup of vinegar or lemon juice and the same of borax, and then rinse well.
● Lay a new shower curtain outside in bright sunshine for a few hours to remove the odour that asthmatics may find an irritant. Alternatively, buy biodegradable cotton shower curtains, which have less odour.
● Consider buying "mould-free" shower curtains. These are impregnated with mould-retardant chemicals.

Towels

● Dry towels and bath mats in a tumble drier or outside, rather than over radiators, to prevent an increase in humidity inside.

Air fresheners

● Avoid using chemical air fresheners in the bathroom, which can irritate sensitive airways, or try the following gentle alternatives:
● One quarter cup of white vinegar, or a bowl of cat litter, set high up on a shelf will effectively deodorize the room.
● If you can tolerate sprayed products, dissolve 1 teaspoon of baking soda and 1 teaspoon of lemon juice completely in 2 cups of hot water. Place in a spray bottle and use as you would an air freshener.
● A bowl of pot pourri is very effective, but the odour may provoke respiratory symptoms in some allergic people.

CHANGES TO MAKE

Essential

● Keep the door shut during and after bathing or showering to prevent water vapour escaping into the rest of the house.
● Open a window after using the bathroom, or install a powered extractor that runs for a pre-set time to remove moisture.
● Replace carpeting with a hard-surface floor.

Desirable

● If necessary, treat any areas of mould with a mould-inhibitor.
● Replace perfumed products with scent-free ones if you are sensitive to strong odours.

CLEANING TIMETABLE

Daily

● Wipe dry all areas of condensation after using the bathroom.
● Dry the bathroom floor after every use.
● Clean the toilet and disinfect it overnight.
● Dry the sink and bath after every use in cockroach-prone parts of the world.

Weekly

● Damp dust or vacuum surfaces, such as skirting (base) boards and windowsills.
● Wash the floor. Keep the window open or the extractor (exhaust) on until it dries.
● Wash out toothbrush holders or beakers.

Every 3–6 months

● Wash any curtains (drapes) at 56°C/ 133°F or above. Add mite-killing benzyl benzoate to materials washed at lower temperatures.
● Treat the shower curtain with mould inhibitor, if necessary.

TOILETRIES

Cosmetics, or toiletries, include soap, shampoo, toothpaste, skin cleansers and moisturizers, eyeshadows, lipsticks, nail varnishes, hair colorants and styling agents, fragranced products (such as deodorants, aftershaves, and perfumes), sun-screens, and self-tanning preparations. Any of these products could cause either irritant or allergic contact reactions.

Irritant reactions

An irritant reaction to cosmetics is most likely in people with a tendency toward allergy (either themselves or in their family), or in people with light-coloured skins. Common symptoms that a cosmetic is having an irritant effect include:

● Scaling

● Redness and associated itching

● No tendency of symptoms to spread beyond the site of application of the cosmetic

Irritant reactions are more likely to occur where the outer layer of the skin is thinnest – such as on the eyelids or backs of the hands – or where the skin is covered – between the fingers or under rings. In general, an irritant reaction is a minor problem that

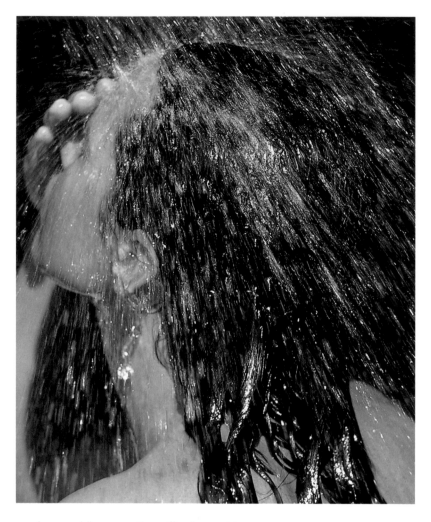

resolves rapidly once the offending agent is removed from contact.

Severe irritant reactions are rare and most often occur at the hairdressers, where a very alkaline

After showering or bathing, apply emollients generously to your skin if you have eczema. These help to keep the skin in good condition, so that it is less likely to develop the complaint.

substance, such as a hair dye or perming solution, has been allowed to come into contact with the skin. When at home, avoid hand contact with shampoos and hair products by using lightweight polythene gloves (as used by hairdressers) if you have sensitive skin or eczema. Don't apply hair lotion, hair cream, or dyes with your bare hands and avoid mousses and hair gels.

If you feel even a slight stinging sensation immediately following the

---

WHAT DOES THE LABEL MEAN?

"Hypoallergenic" commonly appears on cosmetic and skin-care products. "Hypo" simply means "less" or "decreased" and, for example, most cosmetics labelled as "hypoallergenic" will be fragrance-free. Since fragrances are an important cause of skin contact allergy, a cosmetic that does not contain any fragrance is less likely to cause an allergic reaction.

Another commonly used form of wording on labels is "suitable for sensitive skin". Approximately 20–30 percent of people consider that they have "sensitive skin". The phrase has no legal definition, but is often taken to mean that the product is suitable for use by those likely to experience a non-specific reaction, such as redness or itchiness, to a product.

use of a particular cosmetic, take it as a sign that you should consider discontinuing its use.

Contact reactions

An allergic contact reaction involves an immune response to a chemical in the cosmetic, which is most likely to be a preservative of some type. Contact dermatitis occurs where the skin has come into contact with an allergen; a secondary spread may occur if you then touch other parts of your body with hands contaminated with that allergen.

Preservatives are among the most potent allergens found in cosmetics, with the best preservatives often making the strongest allergens.

The chemicals used to make fragrances are another common source of allergens. About 10 percent of people investigated for eczema-like skin conditions are found to be sensitive to fragrances. Other cosmetic allergens include hair dyes and the resin found in nail varnish.

Choosing a product

In general, cosmetics are relatively simple formulations modified with "extras" for marketing. There are many well-priced, non-fragranced products suitable for sensitive skins. Bear in mind that a well-marketed, expensive

Use non-perfumed soaps or cleansing oils in the bath. With children prone to eczema, use only specially prepared bath oils.

product is not necessarily a well-tolerated one. If you are choosing a product for an eczema sufferer, manufacturers may provide samples.

SKIN CARE FOR ECZEMA SUFFERERS

Skin care, especially the use of moisturizing emollients, is a key element in easing the symptoms of eczema and helping the skin to heal. Contrary to popular belief, bathing often can be helpful, since it adds moisture to the skin. However, you must add bath oils formulated for eczema rather than ordinary bubble bath, which has a drying effect. After bathing, it is important to apply emollient to retain skin moisture.

In the bath
● Use non-perfumed soaps or cleansing oils. Only add bath oil that is especially made for eczema sufferers to the water.
● Pat the skin dry – don't rub – with a towel.

● Apply emollients liberally after bathing. Whereas corticosteroid creams should be used only as directed by your doctor, there is no limit on the amount of emollient that can safely be used.

Applying creams and emollients
● Keep your fingernails short and wash your hands carefully before applying creams or emollients to an eczema sufferer. Gently massage only small amounts of cream at a time into the skin using a light, circular motion.
● Encourage absorption and discourage scratching after treatment by bandaging the affected area with sterile cotton gauze. With a child sufferer, make sure that the child's

fingernails are kept short. Use an emery board to file nails down to the finger pads.
● Consider wet-wrapping children with very bad eczema at night. The child is covered in emollient before wrapping in wet bandages, but keep thumbs out to make it easier for the child to pick things up.
● Use emollients on a regular basis to keep the skin moisturized. Use them liberally and frequently, even when the skin is apparently free of eczema. The skin's resistance will be lowered for at least four to five months after the eczema appears to have healed.
● Lanolin-free emollients and bath oils are available for those allergic to this substance.

The Ideal Home Office

As the 21st century unfolds, more and more of us will find ourselves working from home. The move from company site to home office often entails converting a room into a work area. But even a traditional office worker may need a study at home reserved for work-related items, such as a computer.

If you are working from home, the home office becomes increasingly crucial as a factor in your general health. The importance of taking breaks outside the house cannot be over-emphasized, or you may find that days could go by without you ever setting foot beyond your front door. In these circumstances, the overall home environment will have an enormous impact on your health.

For allergy sufferers, it is worth looking back at *The Ideal Bedroom* and *The Ideal Living Room* (see pp. 80–3 and 90–3), since many of the allergy-inducing factors discussed there apply equally to the home office.

The main reservoirs of dust mites in the office will be the carpet and any fabric-upholstered furniture, such as your desk chair. The same guidelines apply: keep humidity low, minimize clutter, keep walls smooth, and buy streamlined furniture so that any dust that does collect is easy to clean. As well, some equipment may produce undesirable emissions, such as the solvents in correcting fluid and ozone emitted by electrical equipment. In addition, poorly designed equipment – such as chairs and desks – lighting, and ventilation can all be sources of physical stress leading to health problems such as repetitive strain injury.

Walls
● Use paint or paper with a washable, non-textured finish. Smooth walls collect less dust and are easier to keep clean.
● Damp-dust picture rail, dado rail, or furniture surfaces weekly to prevent the build-up of dust.
● Consider removing dado or picture rails, if any, if you are undertaking repair work on the walls.

Bookshelves
● Keep books on shelves behind glass doors so that they do not collect dust.
● Avoid storing piles of books, old newspapers, and magazines in the office (or anywhere else in the home). These will absorb moisture and encourage the growth of mould. Throw away any books or papers that smell at all damp or mildewy. Even if you dry them out, they may still retain mould spores.

Office chairs
● Avoid soft-upholstered, padded office chairs. A leather-upholstered chair is a better option, as any dust that collects on it can easily be cleaned away. You are likely to spend most of your time in the office sitting on your chair, so pay particular attention to choosing the right type.
● Take regular breaks if you are spending long periods at the computer keyboard to help avoid repetitive strain injury (RSI).
● Make sure that your chair is properly adjusted as general aches and strains are often caused by badly adjusted furniture. When using a keyboard, your forearms and hands should be level with the keyboard.

Flooring
● Install hard surface flooring, such as vinyl, linoleum, solid wood, or wood laminate, in preference to wall-to-wall carpets.

Ornaments
● To avoid a build-up of dust in the office, keep awards, mementoes, and ornaments to a minimum. Any you want to keep near you should be displayed behind glass doors – not on open shelves or on walls.

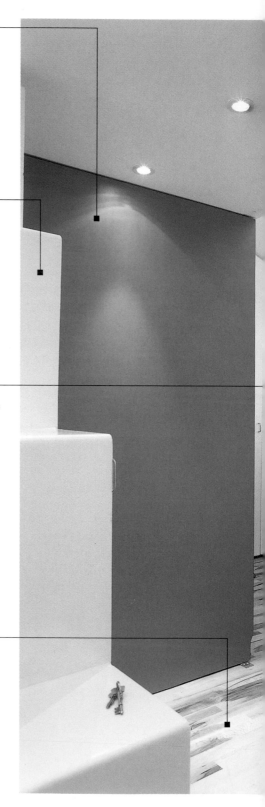

Windows
● Consider using a portable air-filtering unit, fitted with an HEPA filter (see p. 58), if you are a pollen suffer and need to keep the office windows shut during the worst of the pollen season.

● Position computer screens where they will not catch reflected light from windows.
● Use an air-conditioner if necessary in hot, humid weather, but bear in mind that it will not replace indoor air with fresh outside air.

Electrical equipment
● Turn off computers, photocopiers, and laser printers when they are not in use for any length of time, as this type of equipment gives off ozone. In a badly ventilated room where a photocopier, in particular, is running, ozone concentrations can build up to potentially harmful levels. Ozone may worsen allergic symptoms. Check with an allergy association for advice on an approved ozone remover for office use. If possible keep photocopiers in a separate, well-ventilated space.
● Take ease of cleaning into account when purchasing new equipment – smooth surfaces with few awkward corners collect less dust and are easier to clean.
● Use clear, protective dust-covers on computer keyboards. Fine-mesh conductive screens are available for monitor screens. These reduce static electricity, which tends to attract dust particles.

Office furniture
● Treat board-based furniture with caution (see p. 71). Like all products made from board, office furniture made from this material emits formaldehyde. Choose board furniture sealed with a plastic laminate veneer, since this will reduce formaldehyde emission. Avoid exposed board surfaces.
● Choose furniture made from stainless steel, plastic, or solid wood if possible. Be aware that modern furniture is often made of a wood veneer covering a board product.
● Keep office furniture, no matter what it is made from, to the essentials. This minimizes a dust build-up and makes cleaning easier.
● Allow space for the circulation of air behind furniture and storage units to prevent cold spots and mould growth.
● Use waste baskets made of metal or plastic. These are easier to clean than woven cane or fabric types.

Heating
● Consider installing radiant heating. This stirs up less dust than forced-air radiators.
● Turn down the thermostat on your office heating to help to control the mite population. Remember that heat is also generated by electrical office equipment.

CHANGES TO MAKE

Desirable
● Change fabric-upholstered office chairs for ones covered in vinyl or leather.
● Make sure that the office has effective ventilation.
● Put a photocopier in a separate, well-ventilated room because of the ozone it generates.

Optional
● Turn down the temperature to discourage dust mites.
● Replace wall-to-wall carpets with a hard surface floor.
● Replace curtains with blinds.

CLEANING TIMETABLE

Daily
● Wipe or vacuum hard surface floors and any cotton rugs.
● Vacuum the carpet if one is fitted, particularly the area around your armchairs and sofa (couch).
● Empty the waste basket daily and remove any left-over food or drinks, to avoid encouraging cockroaches (or mould).

Weekly
● Vacuum your chair, furniture surfaces, ornaments, windowsills, picture rails, and mouldings, or wipe surfaces over with a damp (not wet) cloth or dust-attracting cloth.
● Tidy away clutter from finished projects or tasks.
● Use vacuum attachments to clean office equipment thoroughly. Some vacuums have keyboard attachments.

Every 3–6 months
● Wash curtains (drapes) or wipe down blinds (shades).
● Wash cotton rugs.

The Ideal Conversion

As an alternative to moving house when more space is required, perhaps to create a home office or a room for a new baby, many people decide to convert their attic (loft) or basement. As when building a new home (see pp. 116–17), this is the perfect time to install measures that are both low-allergen and energy-efficient.

Any conversion work creates huge amounts of dust, which can be a particular problem for those with respiratory allergies or eczema. And when old floorboards are taken up, there is always the risk of mould spores being distributed throughout the home. Allergic individuals who are particularly sensitive to dust or mould may have to consider moving out during the dustiest parts of the work.

You can help to minimize the dust problem by vacuuming numerous times during the day – bear in mind that sweeping just moves the dust into the air, where it can cause even worse problems. In addition, you can try, as far as is practicable, to seal off the area being worked on to reduce the amount of dust and fumes penetrating into the rest of the home. As well as closing internal doors, tape up their edges, or hang plastic curtains at strategic points between the conversion work and the rest of the home.

Using a dehumidifier will help to dry out new plaster and concrete and remove some of the moisture that evaporates from these materials (for up to a year after application); and paying particular attention to ventilation will help to reduce the odours of new paint and building materials.

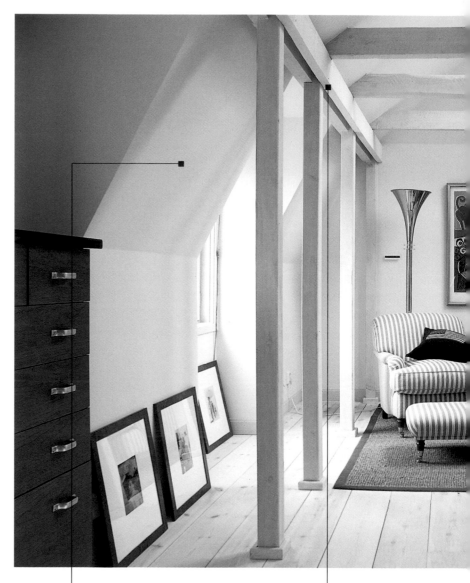

Insulation

● Install foil, polyester, or vermiculite chip insulation in preference to fibre types, such as mineral wool or powdery cellulose insulation. Even low concentrations of insulation particles in the air can irritate the airways and cause coughing and wheezing in some allergic individuals.

Damp

● Check the roof regularly for leaks to stop damp penetration. Blocked gutters will overflow, causing water to saturate the ground around the building and potentially allowing damp into basement foundations.

Timber treatment

● Handle timber treatments carefully to avoid skin contact or breathing in the fumes. Otherwise, they may irritate the skin and mucous membranes, and cause headaches, dizziness, and nausea. Many of the wide range of approved formulations to protect wood from insect or fungal attack contain potentially toxic chemicals and are also often dissolved in VOCs (see pp. 68–9).
● Consider moving out of the home until all odour has disappeared should wood treatment ever become necessary if you have severe asthma or rhinitis. Choose water-based preservatives if possible, as these contain lower levels of VOCs.

Lighting
● Uplighters are useful where you have a sloping ceiling that makes installing recessed ceiling lighting difficult. Uplighters produce a low-glare lighting effect, but they do require more frequent dusting than recessed fittings.

● Consider using recessed light fittings that have no perforations and a tight seal between the light and ceiling. This eliminates air leakage around the fitting, preventing condensation and energy loss.

Windows
● Install double- (secondary-) glazed, high-efficiency windows to reduce condensation and improve energy efficiency.
● Consider windows made with retractable blinds (shades) internal to the window.
● Position the windows strategically to maximize the use of natural light.

Soft furnishings
● Choose leather and vinyl furniture in preference to fabric-upholstered types. Any fabric-upholstered furniture should have removable covers washable at temperatures high enough to kill mites.
● Ensure cushions (pillows) have washable covers or consider putting on an inner anti-mite barrier cover. After washing dry cushions thoroughly to prevent the growth of mould.

Heating
● Consider radiant heating in the form of panels on the walls or within the skirting (base) board. Underfloor heating provides warmth underfoot for hard surface flooring.
● Avoid forced-air central heating, which may blow dust around the room, as may fan and convector heaters, though this problem will be less important if any dust is kept to a minimum.

Flooring
● Install hard surface flooring (tiles, wood, or linoleum, for example), which does not harbour dust and other allergens.
● Choose short-pile, synthetic carpets in preference to deep-pile wool carpets if you don't want a hard surface floor. Some research indicates that the synthetic, short-pile types are easier to vacuum clean and the static charge may help retain allergens between vacuuming, preventing them from becoming airborne. Once installed, all carpet must be vacuumed regularly to minimize dust mites and allergens.
● Keep the room well-ventilated until the smell of a newly installed carpet wears off. Foam-backed carpet should be avoided because of formaldehyde emission.
● Seal wooden floors, as these are easier to clean than unsealed types with gaps, through which dust may blow up from below.

Duct and vents
● Clean ventilation or air-conditioning ducts out thoroughly to remove any dust or debris that may have entered during the conversion work, or when you are building a new home (see pp. 116–17). Otherwise, fine particles from the debris, which can represent a respiratory irritant, may circulate within the ducts and enter the indoor air through room vents.
● Check external and internal air vents to make sure that these have not become blocked or damaged during the building work. Otherwise, your ventilation or air-conditioning system may not work properly.

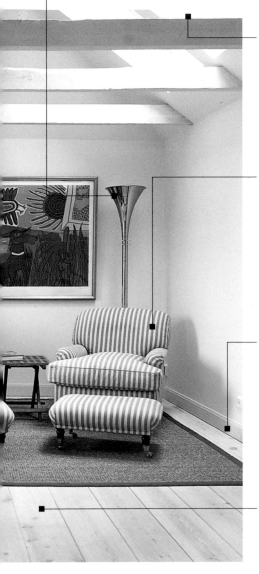

CHANGES TO MAKE

Desirable
● Install a hard surface floor once the carpet needs renewing.
● Replace fabric-covered furniture with leather or vinyl.
● Review the insulation and ventilation in attics (lofts) and basements, as both areas are prone to condensation.

Optional
● Install a humidity meter in a basement to monitor relative humidity.
● Replace curtains or drapes with blinds (shades).

CLEANING TIMETABLE

Daily
● Vacuum hard surface flooring or wipe over with a damp mop or cloth.
● Vacuum carpet or rugs if the room is used daily.
● Damp-dust ornaments and furniture surfaces if the room is used daily.

Weekly
● Damp-dust awkward surfaces, such as on the tops of closets, skirting (base) boards, wall mouldings, rails, and light fittings.
● Polish furniture using non-scented products if you find that fragrances irritate your respiratory system.

Every 3–6 months
● Wash curtains (drapes), if you have them, or wipe down blinds (shades) with a damp cloth.
● Remove and wash covers of fabric-upholstered furniture to remove dust mites and allergen.
● Clean carpets to kill dust mites, but vacuum thoroughly afterwards to remove the dead mites and allergen if necessary.

ALLERGIC FACTORS

Dust, condensation, and mould are commonly found in poorly ventilated and unheated basements, creating problems that can affect the health of everybody in the house. Whether or not you intend to convert an existing basement into a living area, it is still important to treat it as part of the living environment because of the significant impact it can have on the general air quality in the home.

A damp basement is a constant source of moisture, increasing relative humidity throughout the home. The damp also creates favourable conditions for mould. In addition, the dust that builds up in a little used basement inevitably finds its way, through cracks in the floors or walls, into the rest of the home.

Unless you are prepared to improve ventilation and insulation in a damp basement, it might be better to seal it off from the rest of the home. However, if you want to retain easy access, then it is important to find and then correct the causes of any damp.

Solving the problem of damp

Depending on the causes and severity of the damp, you may have to make structural improvements, such as installing a new floor incorporating a moisture or vapour barrier, or building a new inner masonry wall that can be sealed and insulated. If structural alterations are not required, or are prohibitively expensive, an alternative is a portable dehumidifier or air-conditioning unit (see pp. 58–9) to help keep the basement dry. If the damp problem is localized to, say, the inside of a closet, containers of dessicant crystals may help to reduce humidity and, therefore, the potential for mould growth. Electric storage heaters may also help to keep the basement warmer and less humid.

Rugs or carpeting should not be put down over a concrete floor unless it incorporates a moisture or vapour barrier. The difference in temperature between the ground and the basement will cause condensation to form. This may migrate through the floor itself, causing mould to grow on the underneath of any floor covering.

Don't ignore the obvious – some of the commonest reasons for damp in a basement are a leaking appliance, such as a washing machine, or a slow leak from a water pipe.

This utility room has several low-allergen features: streamlined furniture fitting to the ceiling; a lack of cluttered surfaces; and a tumble drier vented to the outside.

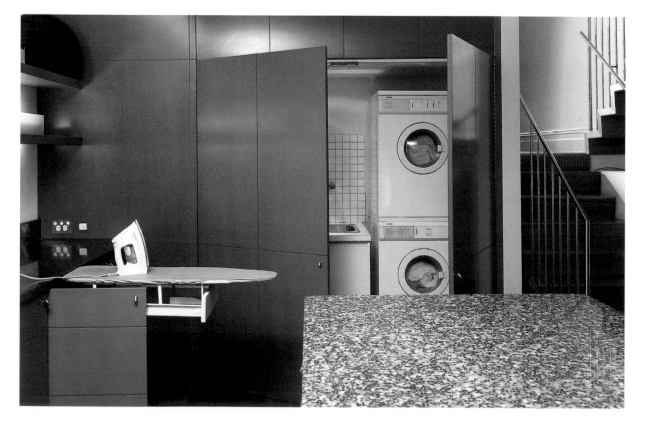

SUCCESSFUL BASEMENT AND ATTIC (LOFT) STORAGE

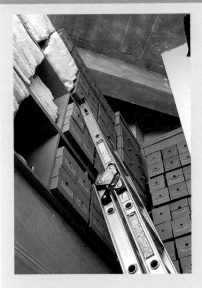

Store items in dry, well-ventilated conditions to protect them from mould. Watch out for cold spots, where air is poorly circulated, as this may encourage condensation.

If your basement or attic is intended for storage, make sure the room is both dry and properly ventilated to prevent condensation and mould growth. Keeping items dry also depends on making sure that the room is properly insulated, as well as preventing damp in a basement, or leaks from a roof, entering the attic.

In a poorly ventilated and unheated basement, the temperature and relative humidity will vary depending on the temperature inside the home and the ground temperature. This will sometimes mean that the relative humidity is high in the basement, resulting in condensation and favourable conditions for mould growth. Once established, mould will colonize almost any item, including files, books, furniture, magazines, and clothing.

Insulation

Foil, polyester insulation or vermiculite chips are preferable to fine and powdery fibre-type insulation. There is also low-odour spray-foam insulation, which is safe for the home environment within 24 hours of application.

Although insulation should be sealed completely from the interior environment, fibres or particles may work their way through cracks in walls or ceilings and enter the air. Even low concentrations can act as an irritant, causing symptoms such as coughing and wheezing in some allergic individuals.

Urea-formaldehyde foam insulation (UFFI) should not be used and has already been banned in many countries. It contains high levels of urea-formaldehyde resin that out-gas formaldehyde into the air for a many months after installation.

A weather-proof roof

Check your roof regularly for leaks, especially after stormy weather that may have dislodged tiles or slates. Also, make sure that gutters and downpipes (downspouts) are not blocked and are working efficiently, otherwise excess water will run off the roof, saturating the outside walls and surrounding ground and leading, potentially, to penetrating damp in both the attic and basement. Mould is likely to grow in gutters blocked by fallen leaves, and a poorly drained flat roof may also harbour mould. Whenever your roof is being repaired, the potential exists for huge quantities of mould spores to be released, causing problems for mould allergy sufferers. Sensitive individuals may need to move out during repairs.

Problems with basement rooms

A basement is most often converted into a utility room. If you want to use this space as a laundry area, install an extractor (exhaust) fan to exhaust excess moisture. Tumble driers should always be vented to the outside, no matter what room they are installed in. Some heat-recovery devices are available that recirculate hot air from the dryer back into the house. However, they are not recommended, since they are unlikely to filter out sufficiently very fine airborne particles.

There is always a possibility of a washing machine leaking or a freezer defrosting, causing some degree of flooding. To forestall problems, the floor of a basement utility room should incorporate a drain to remove any water spills that may occur. If a flood does occur, use a portable dehumidifier to help dry it out.

Boilers or furnaces are sometimes located in basements. A balanced-flue gas boiler ensures that the air used for combustion is drawn from the outside, rather than from inside the room, and that all the flue gases are exhausted outside. This eliminates the need for extra ventilation and relieves you of any worry about escaping combustion by-products mixing with the air inside. Gas condensing boilers are much more efficient than conventional types as they extract heat from the flue gases, which would otherwise be lost to the outside air. Some models are 98 percent efficient compared with conventional boilers, which are about 70 percent efficient (*see pp. 50–9*).

Basements as guest or recreation rooms

It is important to maintain background heat in basements converted to living spaces that are only occasionally used. Even low-level heat will help prevent condensation and mould growth. It may be tempting to furnish basements used as play or recreation rooms with secondhand, cast-off sofas or couches, but these are likely to be full of dust mites and allergen, unless upholstered in leather or vinyl.

Outside The Home

Although many of the allergies that people suffer from are triggered by factors found inside the home, there are some practical steps you can take to improve the wider environment – at your child's school, for example, or in the workplace – in order to minimize the threat posed by eczema, asthma, hay fever, and similar allergic diseases. Of course, you will not have the same degree of control outside the home, but you can often adapt your knowledge about allergy triggers and irritants in the home to these other situations. It may mean, if appropriate, that you make sure your child takes preventative medicine before going on, say, a nature walk or handling the class guinea pig, or you could ensure that only non-perfumed products are used to clean your office.

One of the real danger areas outside the home the allergy sufferer has to consider is the garden. The obvious triggers here are pollen, mould spores, and contact allergens. But there are many ways to minimize or even to prevent these allergies. Strategies range from the careful siting of compost bins to planting only low-allergen specimens (see p. 138). Compared with asthma and hay fever, however, it is far easier to prevent skin allergies simply by avoiding specific plants, but having a pollen or mould allergy does not necessarily make the garden forbidden territory.

Other environments found outside the home that allergy sufferers need to consider carefully include the car and garage, vacation destinations, and visiting other people's houses.

Compost
● Use a closed system of compost making, rather than an open heap, to prevent the escape of fungal spores into the air.
● Turn the compost heap regularly to constantly bring fresh material into contact with the air, and so prevent any fungus establishing itself.
● Don't allow an allergy sufferer to turn the compost or to spread it on the garden.
● Avoid areas of the garden where compost has recently been spread if you are an allergy sufferer.

Children's play areas
● Lay rubber tiles, like those used in playgrounds, instead of grass, if children have grass allergies. The tiles can be cleaned with a garden hose to remove dirt, pollen, fungal spores, and animal waste. Check first that your child is not allergic to rubber (latex).
● Another alternative to grass is the artificial turf used for some tennis courts and football fields.
● Lay non-staining sand to a depth of 30cm/12in over coarse gravel as an allergen-free play area. Fence the area off to exclude cats.

Lawns
● Replace lawns with low-growing ground-cover plants, such as *Vinca minor*, which do not produce pollen.
● If you want to retain a lawn, cut the grass often to keep it short and so prevent it producing flowers and, therefore, pollen.
● Avoid strimmers – these may cause sap to fly up and on to your skin.
● Remove all grass cuttings left behind by a lawn mower.
● Do not walk barefoot if contact with grass causes eczema and urticaria.

Flooring
● Use an easy-to-clean hard surface floor in any room giving access on to the garden. Vinyl, linoleum, solid wood, or glazed tiles all allow you to remove dirt, pollen, fungal spores, grass cuttings, and animal waste that either blow in through open doors or are walked in on the soles of your shoes. Insisting that shoes are removed before coming into the house is a sensible precaution.

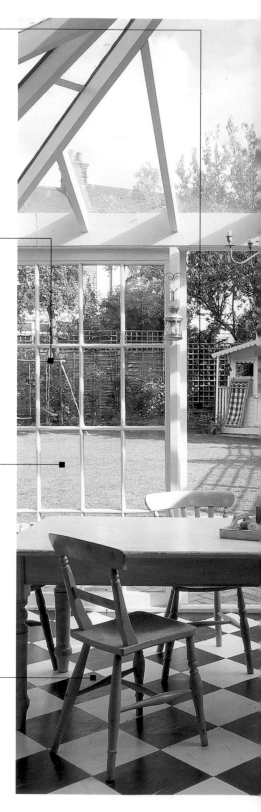

Garden chemicals

● Avoid applying herbicides by using ground-cover plants and low-allergen mulches to deter weeds.
● Use disease-resistant plants, and choose species that thrive naturally in your soil.

● Spray aphids and other pests with liquid soap and water and then wipe them off.
● An effective slug trap is a jar of beer sunk into the ground. A mulch of coarse gravel sometimes deters snails and slugs.

Hedges

● Avoid hedging plants, such as Leyland cypress, that may cause dermatitis, and others, such as privet (*Ligustrum*), that can provoke asthma and hay-fever symptoms.
● Choose closely branched hedging plants, which collect less dust, pollen, and fungal spores.
● Replace hedging with a fence covered with a low-allergen climbing plant, such as a non-scented honeysuckle (*Lonicera*).

Plants

● Avoid strongly scented plants – these are much more likely to cause asthma or hay-fever problems in susceptible people than lightly scented specimens and so should be avoided, especially near seating or play areas.
● Don't plant aromatic herbs, which release their aroma (essential oils) only when they are crushed, anywhere near garden paths, where they may be walked on accidentally. Plant them out of the way in raised beds.
● Reconsider the use of ferns in the garden, as there is some evidence that fern spores cause hay fever in susceptible people.

Conservatories or porches

● Treat a garden room as part of the home, since it will contribute to the quality of the air in the house.
● Install double- (secondary-) glazing to prevent condensation and inhibit moulds.
● Consider installing underfloor heating if building a new conservatory or garden room. This heating system stirs up little dust.
● Choose plants that need little watering and add a top layer of gravel to any exposed soil to inhibit mould. Plants increase general humidity in the home, and so encourage mould growth and dust mites.
● If many plants are present, open windows or consider using a dehumidifier to control humidity.

Garden room furniture

● Avoid soft-upholstered furnishings, but also bear in mind that the traditional wicker and cane furniture commonly found in garden rooms can be difficult to clean.

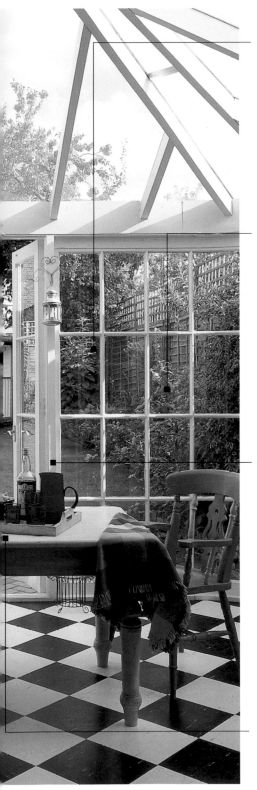

SKIN ALLERGIES

Remove all plants known to be skin allergens or irritants. However, if you do want to grow some of these plants in your garden, take the following precautions:
● Plant problem specimens at the back of a bed or border, well away from paths, to avoid accidental contact.
● Avoid any contact with plants, such as rue (*Ruta*), that cause photodermatitis on hot, sunny days. Photodermatitis results from exposing the skin to a plant in bright sunlight. Brief contact may be enough to cause severe blistering lasting for several weeks.
● Wear a long-sleeved shirt or blouse to protect your arms.
● Wear trousers (pants) rather than a skirt or shorts, particularly when strimming, to protect legs from flying sap.
● Wear a hat to protect your ears, forehead, and scalp.
● Always wash your hands and any exposed skin immediately after a gardening session.

If a plant does irritate your skin:
● Wash the area well with plenty of water and avoid exposing the skin to sunlight for a day or two.
● Try not to rub or scratch the affected area of skin.
● Seek medical advice if the irritation becomes worse.

Knowing your allergy pattern allows you to take precautions:
● Find out what triggers your allergy.
● Keep a daily diary listing your symptoms, their severity, and the weather conditions.
● Use your personal allergy pattern to help you decide when, and in what weather, you can work without problems in your garden.

ALLERGIC TRIGGERS AND IRRITANTS

Allergy sufferers may need to take a range of precautions once they move outside the home.

Bees and wasps

If you are sensitive to bee and wasp stings, take care when eating fruit or having a sweet drink outside. Don't walk barefoot on grass where bees are feeding on small flowers, stay away from tree trunks or stumps that may house wasp nests, and check the car for bees or wasps before getting in. Finally, stay calm if there is a bee or wasp about – any agitated movement will make an attack more likely.

Mosquitoes and midges

An adverse reaction to mosquito or midge bites could include a slight abnormal swelling in the area of the bite, which may be quite marked in some people and lead to prolonged irritation. These symptoms are eased by antihistamine tablets and by applying an anti-irritant cream.

Avoid places where biting insects breed (commonly near ponds and streams) at times when they are active (often in the evening). If you are about at this time of day, wear a long-sleeved top and trousers (pants) and apply an insect-repellent to any exposed areas of skin, especially your ankles. Repellents often contain powerful chemicals you may want to avoid. If so, try rubbing on white vinegar.

Car (automobile) travel

Modern cars (autos) have pollen filters in the ventilation system and many also have air conditioning, which both filters and cools the air. This may be of help for pollen sufferers, as they can keep the windows closed even during the hottest weather.

On the negative side, however, the distinctive smell found in new vehicles is due to chemicals in the upholstery and other components out-gassing. To help speed up this process, let the car (auto) sit out in the hot sun with the windows down. Wiping down the inside thoroughly with a non-scented cleaner may help to remove some of the odour. Avoid air fresheners if you find that fragrances can be an irritant.

To combat mite allergen, avoid soft-fabric seat covers and cushions (pillows), unless they are washable and can be easily dried, and use rubber (latex) floor mats you can take out and wash. These measures, plus regular vacuuming, should help to keep the dust-mite population in check.

Garages and sheds

Many homes with attached garages face the problem of pollutants, including exhaust emissions and volatile organic compounds (VOCs), passing from the garage into the

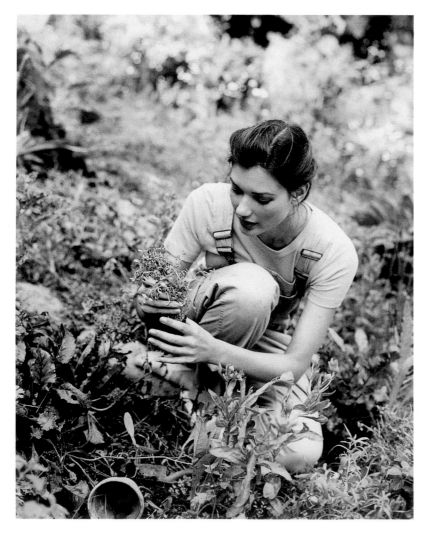

Different parts of the world have indigenous species of trees, shrubs, herbaceous plants, and weeds that are strongly allergenic. Seek advice on plant pollens from a local allergy specialist.

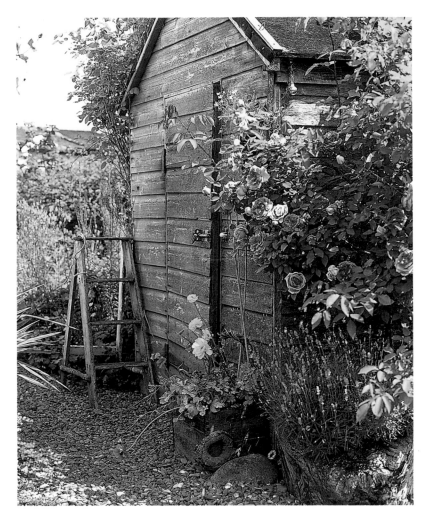

Keep your shed, workshop, or garage tidy and clean to stop dirt and dust accumulating and becoming airborne. Safely dispose of any unwanted or old products that could allow mould or bacteria to develop.

garage door open. Never run your car (auto) in the garage for longer than is strictly necessary – especially if there is a habitable room above it.

Garages and sheds often double up as workshops, and so may contain products with the potential to cause skin or respiratory irritation. Follow the manufacturers' instructions for the storage and use of these products.

Visiting friends

The better you understand your allergy and its trigger factors, the better able you will be to cope with other environments. For example, children with mite allergies intending to sleep over at friends' homes may need to take their own pillows and duvet with them to reduce their risk of worsening their symptoms.

Vacations

People with hay fever and mould allergies may have fewer symptoms during vacations on the coast, as sea breezes contain little pollen; while those sensitive to mites will benefit from a high-altitude vacation in the mountains, where the dust mite is not found.

home. Any connecting door will inevitably allow some polluted air into your home every time it is used.

Carefully draught-proof (weather strip) connecting doors to minimize fume leakage when they are closed, and also seal gaps in walls around pipework passing into your home from the garage. An extractor (exhaust) fan vented to the outside and set to operate for 15–20 minutes after your car has left or entered the garage will help to remove some of the exhaust gases, as will leaving the

---

AVOIDING POLLEN GRAINS AND MOULD SPORES

Pollen grains
- Monitor pollen forecasts, which may be found published in daily newspapers or given out as part of weather forecasts on radio and television.
- If pollen counts are high, remain inside as much as possible. Try to avoid trips out of the home, especially to rural areas where pollen counts are likely to be high.
- Keep windows closed when you are inside. This is most important in the mornings when pollen is being released and in early evening when it is settling back to ground level again.
- Keep windows fully closed in the car (auto) while you are driving.
- Avoid mowing the lawn or raking up leaves. If you must perform these tasks, then use a face mask and eye protectors.
- Wear sunglasses when you are outside, even if only for short periods.

Mould spores
- Avoid going near garden compost heaps – unless they are fully enclosed – fallen leaves, cut grass, barns, and wooded areas.
- Don't walk anywhere near fields when grain harvesting is being carried out.
- Wear a face mask if these places or things cannot be avoided.
- Use low-allergen mulches in the garden.

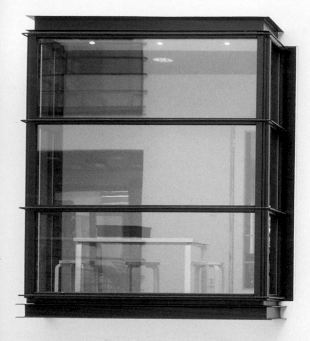
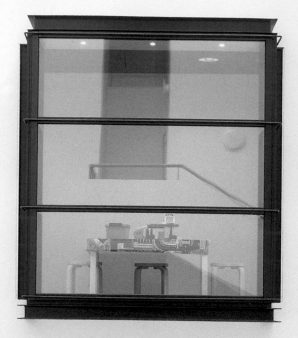
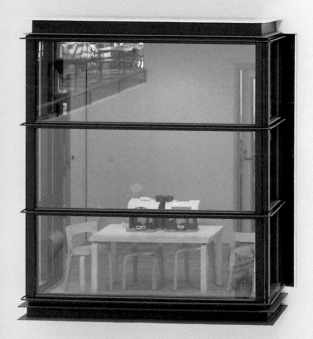
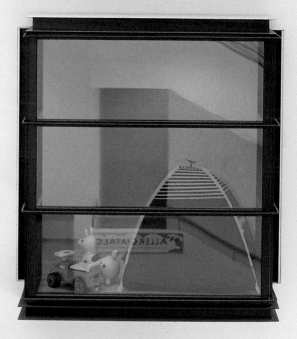
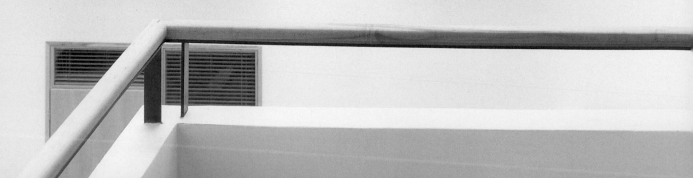

Case Histories

Worldwide, there is increased recognition of the importance of housing and the interior environment to people with asthma and other allergies. Recent building projects include the Allergy House in Helsinki, Finland, the headquarters of the Finnish Allergy and Asthma Federation (see *left*), and a central resource for information on the interior environment and allergy-friendly products to help people alleviate their allergic symptoms. In addition, the Finnish Association of the Pulmonary Disabled, also based in Helsinki, is scheduled to begin building low-allergen homes for families with asthma. Elsewhere in Europe, the municipal housing association of Rotterdam, Holland, is planning 40 homes for low-income families with asthmatic children in Barendrecht, a suburb of Rotterdam. Families will be given support on how to manage their home environment and research will be done on the effects of the new housing on asthma. Other cities across Holland are showing keen interest in Rotterdam's initiative.

In the USA, the American Lung Association has been building its own series of healthy homes since 1993. Over 18 demonstration houses have now been built in 11 states across America to help builders and homeowners make better choices for their health and homes when building, remodelling, and maintaining a home.

Australians have one of the highest incidence of asthma in the world, and here, too, steps are being taken to reduce the disease toll by changing the interior environment. The first case history in this chapter, in Melbourne, Australia, describes the building and design of Sunbury Healthy House in Melbourne (see pp. 118–123), while the second case history shows how the Asthma Victoria Breathe Easy campaign has helped Leisl Wood, a young woman with incapacitating asthma, build her own low-allergen, asthma-friendly home (see pp. 124–127).

Building from scratch

Low-allergen features can be most comprehensively incorporated into a building at the design stage or as part of the renovation of an existing building. While it is true that you can make many changes to the structure and interior of any home to make it more allergen-free, some features, such as installing a mechanical ventilation system with heat recovery or making the building airtight, can be most easily accomplished when building from scratch.

Most of the low-allergen homes that are being built today are also designed to high standards of energy and resource efficiency – making them good for the environment as well as for the people living in them. The basic principles of healthy housing design, as defined by the American Lung Association (ALA), provide a good reference point. An example of these principles in practice can be seen in the first case history, the story of Sunbury Healthy House, Melbourne, Australia (see pp. 118–23).

The overall aim is to create a healthy and comfortable environment, with the emphasis on improving the interior air quality to a standard that we should all expect – not just those with asthma and other allergies.

Designing and building your own home allows you to take location into account, such as building away from busy roads (external pollution) and on dry soil and away from damp valleys, underground springs, or rivers (to avoid damp). It also allows you to make sure you emphasize those low-allergen features specific to your condition. For someone highly sensitive to dust-mite allergen, for example, the main aim would be to create a domestic environment that is inhospitable for the mite. The house will therefore contain leather or vinyl-covered sofas (couches) and chairs, or at least a minimum of fabric-upholstered furnishings, preferably with washable covers; hard surface flooring with washable cotton rugs; a ventilation system to help control relative humidity and interior pollution; and a central vacuum cleaning system to exhaust allergen-containing dust outdoors.

For those highly sensitive to pollen, but not mites, the garden will be particularly significant. Rather than being concerned about carpeting and soft furnishings, the emphasis will be more on low-allergen planting. Those with food allergies may want to make sure that there are plenty of cabinets in the kitchen to store bulk purchases of special foods.

So, if you have decided to build a healthy, low-allergen home, who will help you turn your vision into reality?

Deciding on an architect

There is an increasing number of architects and building consultants specializing in the construction of healthy housing, but as Leisl Wood discovered, in *Case History 2* (see pp. 124–7), a general architect was able to build a low-allergen home for her with help from the Asthma Victoria Breathe Easy initiative.

One of the most important points to bear in mind when deciding on an architect is entirely personal – you will be spending a lot of time with that person, so make very certain that it is somebody with whom you feel able to resolve the disagreements that will inevitably arise.

You may find the following points useful:

- Local architects are likely to have a good understanding of the local conditions that will impact on your specific requirements, such as terrain, orientation, and micro-climate, and even the attitude of local authorities concerning planning and permissions.

- If possible, collect the names of local architects to interview from personal recommendations. Failing this, contact national allergy associations (particularly those with an interest in low-allergen housing), professional bodies and associations, or refer to the advertisements you will find at self-build exhibitions, which are becoming more and more commonplace.

- Make a full list of all the points about your specific low-allergy requirements you want to discuss with each architect.

- At the initial meeting find out how soon the practice could start on your project and the fee structure proposed.

- Before making your final decision, ask for references, preferably for similar work, and follow them up.

Designing your own low-allergy home allows you to emphasize those particular features helpful to your allergic condition, such as hard surface flooring or low-allergen plants in the garden.

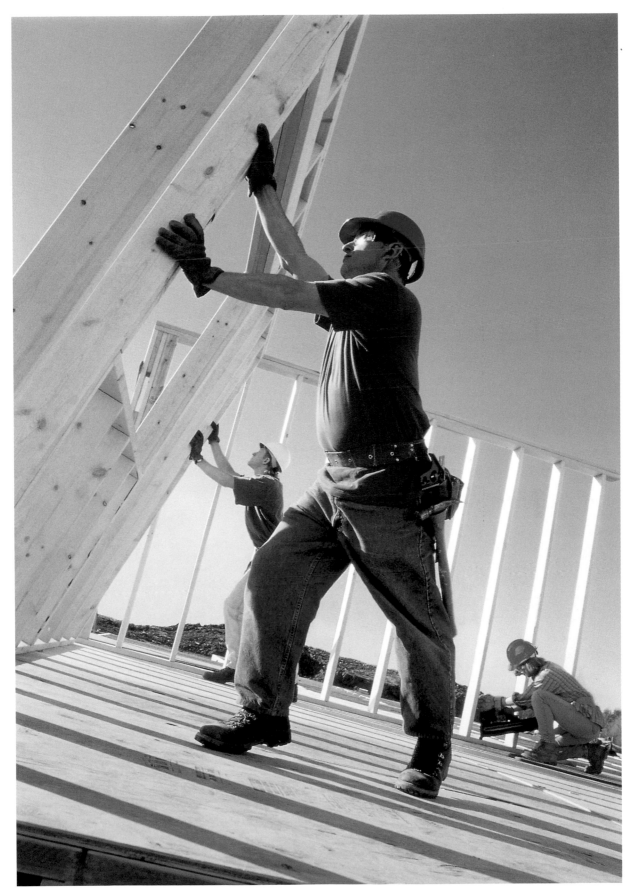

Case History 1

Sunbury Healthy House, Melbourne, Australia, has been designed as a model home for healthy living. It has been built to maximize the interior air quality and energy efficiency by the Australian Healthy House Institute, an organization itself inspired by the healthy housing programme of the American Lung Association (see p. 116). The house has many features that make it suitable for people with allergies, including a mechanical ventilation system that purifies the air and removes excess moisture, and an interior design scheme that discourages the house-dust mite.

However, Sunbury Healthy House is more than just a show home; it is also home to one of the house's designers, Jan Brandjes and his young family, who emigrated to Australia from Canada in 1996. Since moving into Sunbury Healthy House 18 months ago, Jan has seen his children benefit from living in a healthy home environment.

"When we first came to Australia we were living in temporary accommodation," says Jan. "Both my little girls, Annelies and Mollie, soon developed asthma symptoms, having shown no signs of any allergy before. They had to spend a lot of time on a Ventolin pump machine, prescribed by our doctor, to stop them coughing and wheezing at night. Since we moved into Sunbury Healthy House, however, their coughs and wheezing have stopped completely and they haven't once had to use the Ventolin pump. Our little son, Felix, born just a week before we moved in, has shown no signs of asthma."

When Jan moved to Australia, he brought with him more than 15 years' experience of building energy-efficient healthy houses for the Canadian government. Soon after his arrival, he founded the independent Australian Healthy House Institute, together with Bernard Desmoreaux, an Australian building consultant, in the belief that Australians could also benefit from the lessons learned in North America and Europe concerning the building of healthy homes.

At present, most Australians pay little attention to how the structure of their homes affects their living environment. However, attitudes are beginning to change as more people become aware of the importance of interior air quality and its effect on health and well being, especially for those people with allergies.

Between 6 and 7 million Australians (about 41 percent of the total) suffer from allergies. Much of this problem is related to the fact that the centre of Australia is a vast desert, with hot winds blowing dust and allergens, such as ragweed pollen, into the populated coastal areas. Australian homes also have high levels of relative humidity, and this encourages mould growth and mites (see pp. 36–7 and 42–3). Jan and Bernard believe that homes like Sunbury Healthy House are a key part of the answer to improving the life of people with allergies in Australia.

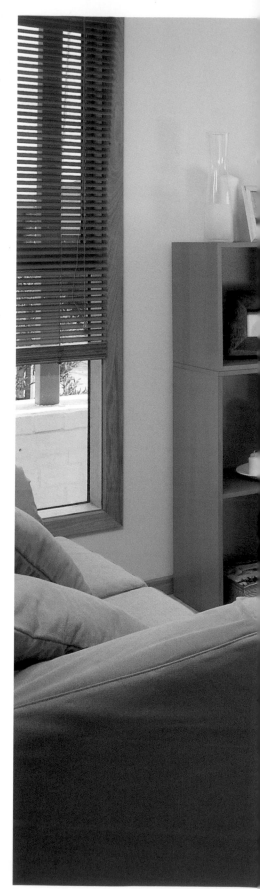

Sunbury Healthy House is a comfortable home. Low-allergen features, such as hard surface flooring with washable rugs, stream-lined furniture and walls, and blinds or shades rather than curtains, also make it a healthy one.

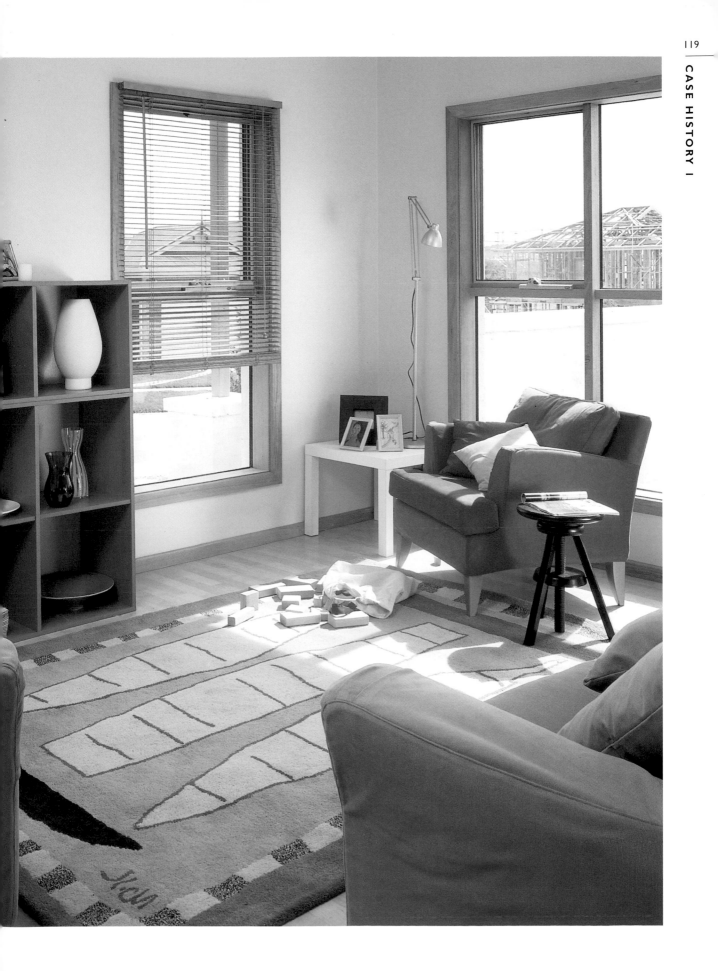

Design principles

The design of the Sunbury Healthy House has been based on the following guiding principles:

- Elimination. There are hundreds of chemicals used in the construction of a typical modern building. Where possible, building products or furnishings containing toxic chemicals have been eliminated.
- Separation. Products containing potentially toxic chemicals or materials, but which are essential in construction, are separated from the interior air by, for example, encasing them in plastic laminate.
- Ventilation. This is considered essential in providing and maintaining good interior air quality. Sunbury Healthy House uses a mechanical ventilation system, which provides adequate amounts of filtered, humidity-controlled air to the whole home, while expelling stale, polluted air.
- Energy efficiency. The energy-efficiency features of Sunbury

Healthy House – insulation, double- (secondary-) glazing, and sealing cracks and holes – have created an airtight house that, in turn, allows control of the interior environment through the mechanical ventilation system. Overall, the Healthy House uses between 50 and 70 percent less energy, compared with the average home meeting the standard housing building regulations.

- Surfaces. As a general design principle, there are very few horizontal surfaces in the house. This prevents dust from collecting and makes the home easier to keep clean and dust-free.

Since it is recognized that building materials and interior design can have a profound effect on the quality of air in the home, Sunbury Healthy House pays particular attention to the construction and materials used in the house. These encompass everything from the types of wood used for the flooring and any

built-in furniture to the paint on walls and the level of insulation installed.

Non-VOC products Paints, sealants, and other coatings used in homes often contain significant quantities of volatile organic compounds (VOCs; see pp. 68–9). These are released into the air as gases after application and may cause respiratory irritation. The products used in the Sunbury Healthy House have been chosen for their low VOC content to minimize the impact on the interior air quality.

Cabinetry materials Wherever possible built-in cabinets and closets have been made of solid wood rather than particle board, which is commonly found in modern homes. Particle board is usually made with glues containing formaldehyde. This is emitted (out-gassed) over time and may cause irritation of the upper respiratory tract and other problems. In Sunbury Healthy House, the kitchen and bathroom cabinets are built with particle board that has been encased in plastic laminate to minimize the escape of formaldehyde. A ventilated shelving system is employed in the wardrobes and laundry areas to discourage mould and house-dust mites.

Flooring Tiles or wooden laminate floors have been used throughout the Sunbury Healthy House. Both of these materials are durable and attractive but, of more importance, they provide clean, non-dust-gathering surfaces that can be regularly maintained without the use of chemical cleaning agents.

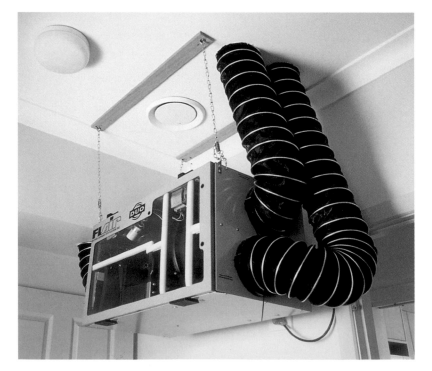

A key part of Sunbury Healthy House is the mechanical ventilation system, which incorporates an energy-recovery device that controls temperature and maintains relative humidity at between 30 and 55 percent.

There is no wall-to-wall carpeting anywhere in the house, and so a major potential reservoir for house-dust mites and mould is removed.

Mechanical ventilation "Natural" ventilation does not guarantee a good supply of fresh air. On calm, windless days, for example, little natural ventilation can occur, and so a mechanical ventilation system makes sure that there is always a healthy rate of air exchange throughout the entire building.

Fresh incoming air is filtered to remove 95 percent of pollen and dust before it is distributed through a sealed duct system into the living and sleeping areas, while moist, stale air is removed at source from the kitchen, bathroom, and laundry areas.

The type of mechanical ventilation system used in the Healthy House gives occupants control over the interior humidity and temperature. This is done with a "dessicant wheel", a high-tech device that ensures that incoming air contains the right amount of moisture and is at the right temperature, in both summer and winter.

Setting the humidity control (humidistat) to between 30 and 55 percent relative humidity prevents the growth of moulds and greatly inhibits the spread of the house-dust mite.

The mechanical ventilation system also gives the occupants an opportunity to protect themselves from allergens originating from outside the home, such as pollen or vehicle exhaust emissions. At times of peak pollen (in the morning and early evening) or pollution levels, the occupants can close up their home and breathe air that has first been passed through the filter in the building's ventilation system.

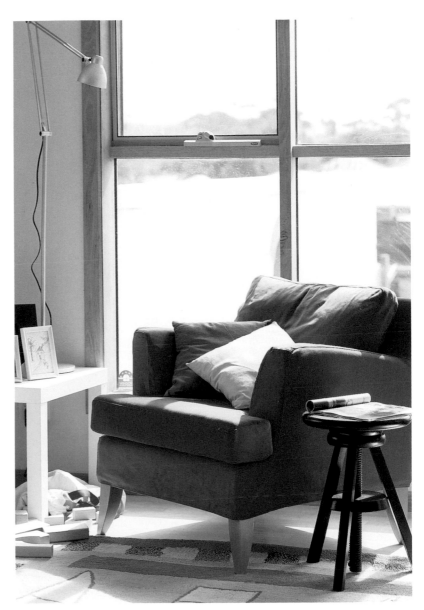

Mechanical ventilation of this type can be installed in an existing home, provided that all cracks and holes in the structure are first sealed. This is done using a foam sprayed from a canister. Once in contact with the air, the foam expands to fill the cracks and sets to become a barrier to the movement of air and heat. The foam sets quickly and its low odour clears within an hour. This treatment restricts air movement into and out of the building to that passing through the ventilation system – provided, of course, that the doors and windows are closed.

Jan and his family have kept fabric upholstery and cushions or pillows to a minimum. Other furniture is streamlined and made of solid wood. This avoids the formaldehyde that would be out-gassed from particle-board products.

Air conditioning (cooling) No cooling is needed in Sunbury Healthy House due to the high insulation specification of the building's envelope (windows, walls, ceilings, doors, and floors), which reduces the movement of heat into and out of the building. The addition of the heat wheel to the ventilation system also reduces cooling and heating requirements.

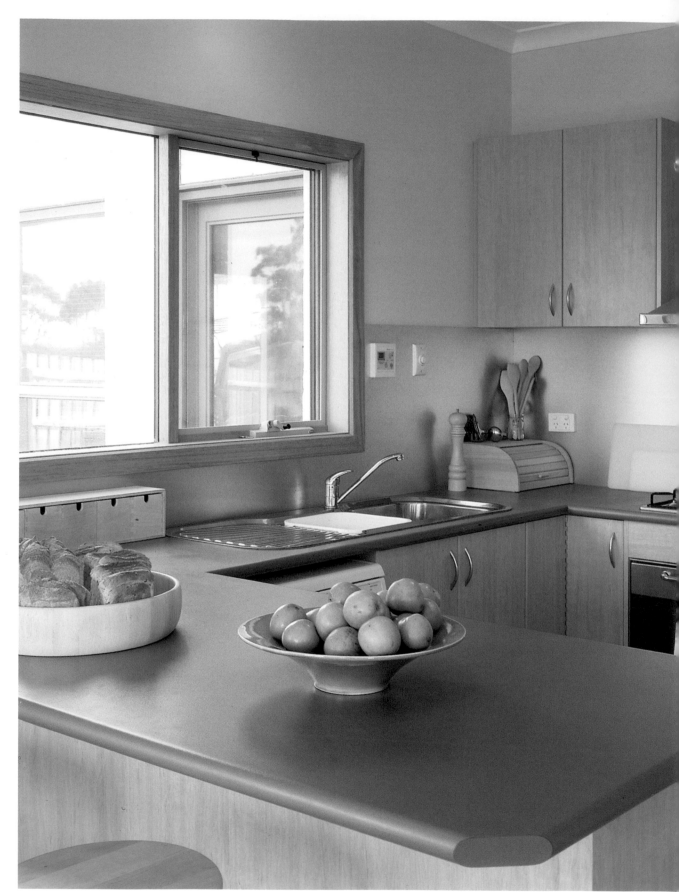

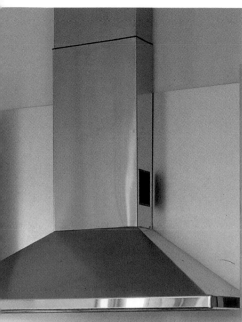

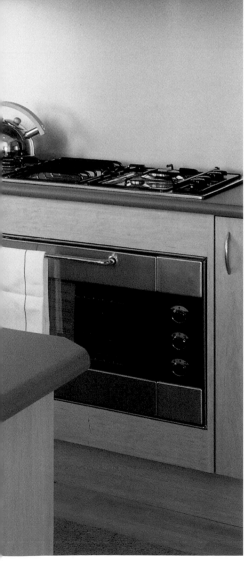

However, if at any time it is decided that an air-conditioning unit is needed to further cool the air, then the advantage of living in a well-sealed, well-ventilated home will immediately become apparent. Because the occupants can rely on their home's ventilation system to move the cooled air around the interior, a smaller air-conditioning unit will be needed than would otherwise be the case.

Insulation The building has been insulated to a very high level. The insulation measures in the house act as a thermal barrier against the movement of heat through the envelope of the house (windows, walls, ceilings, doors, and floors). This degree of insulation helps to regulate the temperature inside the house, thus ensuring that energy is not unnecessarily wasted by leaking out through the building's structure.

Vapour barrier To allow the house's insulation to function effectively, the outside of the building contains a barrier consisting of a breathable plastic membrane. This barrier eliminates the possibility of moisture becoming trapped within the walls and so reduces the potential for wood rot and mould growth.

However, great care must be taken during the installation of this barrier to make sure that it is continuous and properly sealed, otherwise its effectiveness is greatly reduced. This includes sealing all electrical outlets and any plumbing that pierces the external walls.

The particle board used to make the kitchen cabinets is completely encased in plastic laminate veneer to minimize formaldehyde emission. An extractor hood above the range exhausts moisture and cooking smells outside.

Moisture barrier During the construction of the house, a layer of plastic sheeting was used to cover the ground beneath the concrete foundations. This helps to prevent ground moisture from permeating into the house.

Windows and doors The windows are made of high-quality double- (secondary-) glazing, incorporating a low-emissivity coating (a thin, metallic coating that slows down the rate at which glass radiates heat) and non-heat-conductive frames. The thermal efficiency provided by the windows increases comfort and eventually saves enough energy to offset the initial higher installation costs.

All gaps around the windows have to be sealed to minimize air and heat transfer. The preferred sealing method involves an expandable foam material inserted between the window frames and exterior wall frame. Silicone is used for any very small gaps. And all exterior doors are fully weather-sealed and draught-proofed (weather stripped) for comfort and energy-efficiency.

Heating The heating requirements of Sunbury Healthy House are approximately 60 percent lower than those in the average home in the state of Victoria. A high-efficiency, forced-flue gas space heater in the main living area provides a comfortable temperature throughout the whole house during the winter period. The balanced flue used by this type of heating system allows air for combustion to be taken from outside the building, while all the combustion by-products are forced out. By using this type of system, indoor oxygen levels are not compromised and energy efficiency is extremely high.

Case History 2

Australia has one of the worst incidences of asthma in the world. In the state of Victoria 600,000 people out of a population of 4 million have asthma. In an attempt to rectify this situation, the charitable organization Asthma Victoria has developed, in association with electricity supplier Eastern Energy (TXU), the Asthma Victoria Breathe Easy Low Allergy Living Programme, which aims to advise people on reducing their exposure to domestic allergens and irritants.

Working with top architects, Asthma Victoria and Eastern Energy (TXU) have created eight display homes, built in a variety of styles and to suit different budgets, each illustrating a range of asthma-friendly features. These features can be incorporated into any building, preferably at the initial design stage but also as part of a renovation.

Breathe Easy's key features

The Asthma Victoria Breathe Easy Low Allergy Living Programme gives those with asthma and their families specific and practical information about making their homes more asthma friendly. In this way, people are able to identify and reduce domestic sources of allergens and other asthma triggers, thereby helping to create a healthy and comfortable environment.

Ventilation Good ventilation stops the build-up of moisture and fumes. Breathe Easy recommends installing extractor (exhaust) fans, preferably vented to the outside, in the bathroom, kitchen, and laundry, as well as an effective cooker (stove) hood. All rooms should have fixed air vents, and windows and doors should be situated to achieve cross-ventilation.

Flooring All floor surfaces should be easy to clean and discourage mites.

Streamlined cabinets up to the ceiling in this Breathe Easy kitchen are easy to keep dust-free. Electric cooking is preferred; an exhaust hood, vented to the outside, has been installed.

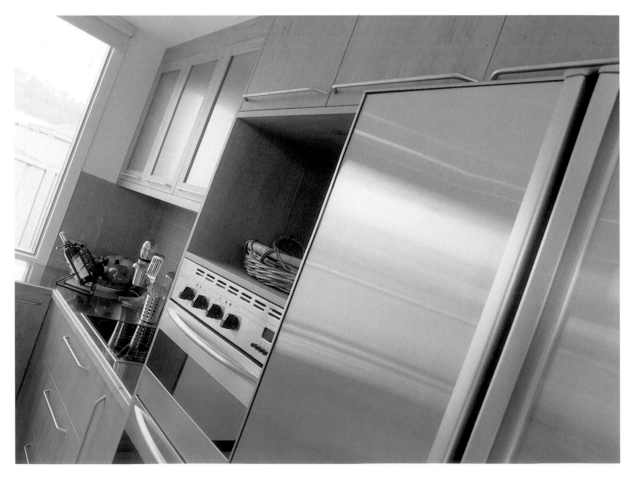

Carpets, therefore, should be removed and be replaced with glazed ceramic tiles, sealed wood or cork, or slate.

Heating Breathe Easy recommends radiant heating (heated tiles in the floor or radiant panels fitted on to walls or ceiling, for example) in preference to other types (such as water-filled radiators or fan heaters). Radiant heating does not collect or circulate dust or produce particles or combustion by-products. Any gas appliances, such as boilers, should be located outside, well away from any air vents, to prevent combustion gases being sucked back inside.

Cooking appliances Electricity is the recommended system, as it does not create combustion by-products. However, an efficient hood over the cooker (stove) is needed to remove the steam produced by cooking pots.

Insulation Foil or polyester insulation does not produce irritant particles that float in the air, where they can be breathed in.

Central vacuum system This has the advantage of removing dust to an external collection bag or bin and avoids the possibility of dust being recirculated inside the home.

Air conditioning Breathe Easy recommends that people with asthma should avoid evaporative systems, in which moisture tends to build up, as there is a risk of mould growth.

Dust prevention Because of the role of the house-dust mite in the prevalence of asthma symptoms, all measures should be taken to prevent the build-up of dust in any part of the

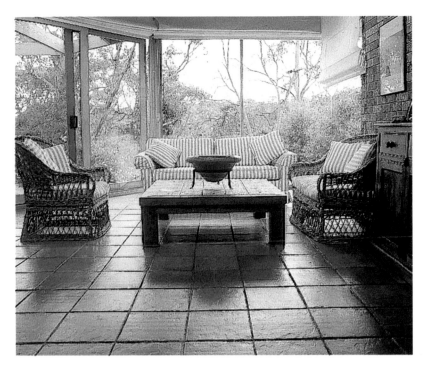

Glazed ceramic tiles have been used in this Breathe Easy living room to discourage dust mites. Other materials you could use include sealed wood, sealed cork, or slate.

home. The most obvious steps to take include the following:
- Build cabinets up to the ceiling, choose flush fittings, and avoid elaborate mouldings
- Add doors to open shelving
- Install easy-clean vertical or roller blinds or shades rather than heavy drapes
- Choose vinyl- or leather-covered upholstery or wooden seats
- Use special dust-mite barrier covers on beds and bedding
- Choose polyester fabrics and fillings that can be hot washed (see p. 83)

Tobacco smoke This is a major trigger and risk factor for asthma, so smoking should be banned inside.

Garden allergens A garden should not increase an asthma sufferer's exposure to pollens and moulds. This is achieved by choosing bird- or insect-pollinated plants and non-pollinating ground cover plants. Rye grass should be avoided and weeds should not be allowed to flower. Weed control can be aided by replacing lawns with paved areas and using pebbles or gravel instead of mould-producing mulch.

Breathe Easy in practice

The story of Leisl Wood and her fight to gain control over her asthma symptoms is an inspirational example of what the Breathe Easy programme is all about. As a result of her experience, Leisl's advice is: "Know what your asthma triggers are and try to eliminate them from your environment. What you cannot remove, simply avoid." Leisl Wood is now 26 years old and has suffered from severe asthma since she was 3 years old. At the age of 19, her asthma became so bad that she gave up her job and returned home to be cared for by her parents, while the doctors battled to get her asthma under control.

Leisl became bedridden and spent increasingly long periods in hospital, up to 3 weeks at a time. During the worst period of her illness, she was taking 70–100mg per day of an oral corticosteroid drug to keep her symptoms at bay. This was increased to a 150mg per day during her hospital stays for severe attacks. These high doses of steroid caused her weight to soar from 65kg (143lb) to 110kg (242lb), but still her asthma was not under control.

Leisl's peak flow readings, which show how well the lungs are functioning, plunged to between 150 and 200 litre/min – a drastic reduction when compared with the predicted normal for Leisl of 49litre/min. She was continually short of breath and had to be helped with tasks as simple as dressing or washing her hair.

But then, two years ago, things began to take a turn for the better. In an effort to improve Leisl's asthma, doctors advised her to try a personal fitness trainer. Exercise is thought to benefit asthma by improving lung function and general fitness. "I was very reluctant, as my asthma is

induced by exercise," said Leisl. "At first, I could do little more than squeeze a stress ball in my hand and raise my legs in the air. Every breath was an effort and I thought the situation was hopeless."

However, Leisl persisted with the training and gradually began to notice strength increasing. As her fitness improved, so did her peak flow reading. Eventually she built up her training to a full daily gym workout and bike programme.

At the same time as undertaking her fitness programme, Leisl also began a special diet. Skin prick tests had determined that Leisl was allergic to a range of substances, such as dust-mite allergen, cat dander, some moulds, pollen, and certain household chemicals. In addition, Leisl was allergic to some foods, including vegetables, oranges, basil, chilli, food colourings, and preservatives. Eliminating these from her diet contributed to the improvement in Leisl's asthma.

At about this time Leisl and her parents heard about the Breathe Easy campaign, run by Asthma Victoria, the Victoria State Asthma Foundation

branch of the national Asthma Foundation of Australia.

Inspired by Breathe Easy's advice, Leisl's parents commissioned a local architect to design a specially adapted low-allergen home for her, right next door to the family home. Here, Leisl would have her independence, while help would be close at hand if needed. Leisl took possession of her house in December 1997.

Two years later, Leisl's symptoms have shown great improvement. Her asthma is now stable and her peak flow reading has climbed to a healthier average of 480litre/min. Her weight has dropped back to a near normal 66kg (145lb), and her medication is much reduced.

Leisl's home is a bright and cheerful bungalow. There are two bedrooms, a large bathroom, and an open-plan kitchen and living area. Its streamlined fittings and uncluttered look give the house a fresh, contemporary feel. The walls, woodwork, and cabinets are all painted with low-odour, asthma-friendly paint. The floors are wood throughout, with only one washable rug, except in the bathroom, which has ceramic tiles. There is no carpet anywhere in the house, which would act as a reservoir for house-dust mites.

Her bedroom has little furniture, just a bed and bedside table. Her clothes are in built-in closets, hung on wire racks that are designed to increase air flow and so discourage house-dust mites. She keeps no ornaments in her bedroom and very few in the rest of her house. Those she does have are displayed in a glass-fronted cabinet. This lack of clutter is

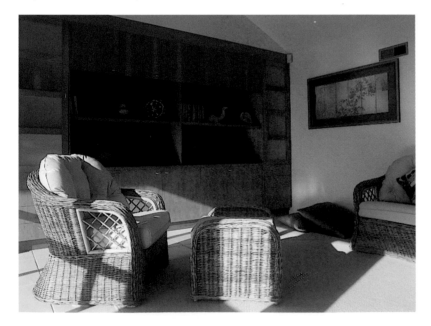

Keep soft furnishings to a minimum if you are unable to replace fabric-upholstered examples with leather or vinyl. Fabric-covered furniture provides the ideal breeding conditions for mites.

designed to make all household surfaces easy to wipe clean of dust.

Nearly all her furniture is made of solid wood with a minimum of the type of detailing that soon becomes a dust trap. No particle board, or other types of board product, has been used in the house, to avoid the emission of formaldehyde gas.

In the living area Leisl has two fabric sofas (couches) covered with throws, which she washes regularly to remove dust mites and mite allergen. Although leather-covered sofas are better than fabric-covered ones, because they are inhospitable to dust mites, leather was beyond her budget.

Venetian blinds or shades have been used throughout instead of curtains. The slats of these blinds are vertical rather than horizontal, and so collect less dust and are easier to clean. They are also made of wipable plastic to discourage mites. The double- (secondary-) glazed windows have no windowsills – ledges and edges of any sort have been kept to a minimum to prevent dust building up.

Heating is provided by electric storage heaters, which radiate heat. Forced-air duct heating systems or fan heaters are not recommended by

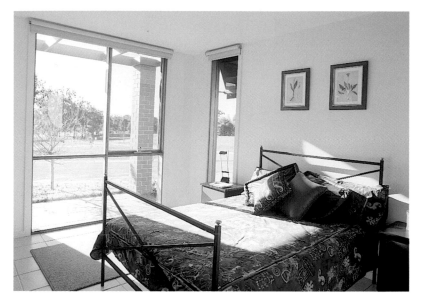

Low-allergen features in the bedroom include a hard surface floor, anti-mite bedding covers, vertical blinds or shades, and a minimum of clutter to collect dust.

Breathe Easy as they stir up dust. And a mechanical ventilation system has been installed that filters out pollen. Leisl is slightly sensitive to pollen but develops pollen-related asthma symptoms (coughing and wheezing) only on windy days. She then closes up her home and relies on the filter in the mechanical ventilation system to prevent the pollen from entering the house. Extractor (exhaust) fans in the bathroom and kitchen remove excess moisture.

The house's asthma-friendly insulation does not release particles or fibres into the air, which might then be breathed in to aggravate Leisl's asthma symptoms. Two layers of insulation have been included to increase energy efficiency and make the home more airtight.

Leisl is careful to use non-fragranced cosmetics and hair products. "I keep to those brands that I know will not trigger my symptoms," she says. "I have to be careful with household products as well. Strong chemicals, especially those with an

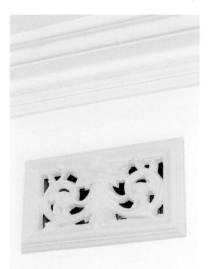

Good ventilation, to avoid a build-up of moisture and fumes, is an essential part of the Breathe Easy programme, and includes fixed air vents in all rooms.

ammonia base, are powerful irritants. I use a few lemon-scented products, which, despite their perfume, seem to cause me no problems."

Leisl used to wear a dust mask when vacuuming. Since moving into her new home, she no longer has to do this, mainly because of the efficiency of the house's central (ducted) vacuum cleaner, which exhausts all the dust and dirt to a container situated outside.

Leisl's recovery means she is now beginning to live life again rather than endure it. She has started a business course by correspondence and has taken up her craft hobbies.

The severity of her asthma has taken its toll, however. She will soon need both hips replaced because of the bone destruction caused by the years of treatment with high levels of steroids. But she remains remarkably buoyant. "Some days are harder than others," she adds, "but I manage. You've got to stay positive."

Reference

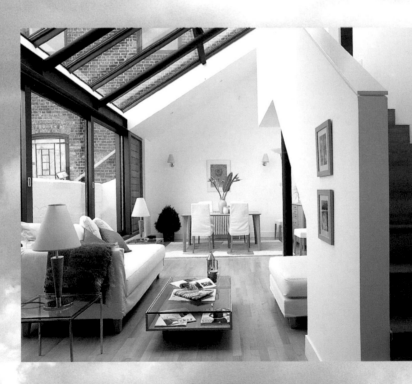

Directory

UNITED STATES OF AMERICA

Organizations

Allergy and Asthma Network/Mothers
    of Asthmatics Inc
2751 Prosperity Ave, Suite 150
Fairfax, VA 22031
Tel: 703 641 9595; Fax: 703 573 7794
Toll-free: 1-800 878 4403
Email: aanma@aol.com
Web: www.aanma.org

Allergy to Latex Education and
    Resource Team (ALERT Inc)
PO Box 13930
Milwaukee, WI 53213
Tel: 262 677 9707; Fax: 262 677 2808
Toll free: 1-888 97 ALERT
Email: alert@execpc.com
Web: www.execpc.com/~alert

American Lung Association
1740 Broadway
New York, NY 10019
Tel: 212 315 8700; Fax: 212 265 5642
Toll-free: 1-900 LUNG USA
Web: www.lungusa.org

American Society of Heating,
    Refrigerating, and Air-Conditioning
Engineers (ASHRAE) Inc
1791 Tullie Circle, NE
Atlanta, GA 30329
Tel: 404 636 8400; Fax: 404 321 5478
Web: www.ashrae.org

Asthma and Allergy Foundation
    of America Inc
1233 20th Street, Suite 402
Washington, DC 20036
Tel: 202 466 7643; Fax: 202 466 8940
Toll-free: 1-800 ASTHMA

Canadian Housing Information Center
(Canada Mortgage and Housing Corp)
700 Montreal Road
Ottawa, Ontario, Canada, K1A OP7
Tel: 613 748 2367

Health House Project
(American Lung Association)
490 Concordia Avenue
St Paul, MN 55103
Tel: 651 227 8014; Fax: 651 281 0242
Email: webmaster@healthhouse.org
Web: www.healthhouse.org

Indoor Air Quality Information
Clearinghouse (IAQ INFOR)
(Environmental Protection Agencies)
PO Box 37133
Washington DC 20013
Tel: 703 356 4020; Fax: 703 356 5386
Toll-free: 1-800 438 4318
Email: iaqinfo@aol.com
Web: www.epa.gov/iaq

National Eczema Association for
    Science and Education
1220 SW Morrison Street, Suite 433
Portland, OR 97205
Tel: 503 228 4430; Fax: 503 224 3363
Toll-free: 1-800 818 7546
Email: nease@teleport.com
Web: www.eczema-assn.org

National Air Duct Cleaners Association
1518 K Street NW, Suite 503
Washington, DC 20005
Tel: 202 737 2926
Web: www.nadca.com
*Professional association of ventilation
system cleaning. Certifies duct-cleaning
companies*

Office on Smoking and Health/Centers
    for Disease Control
Center for Disease Control and Prevention
Mail Stop K-50,
4770 Buford Highway
Atlanta, GA 30341
Toll-free: 1-800-CDC-1311
Web: www.cdc.gov/tobacco
Information on smoking, tobacco, & health

Renee Theodarakis, MA
1080 Glen Cove Avenue
Glen Head, NY 11545
Tel: 516 625 5735
Email: reneetheod1@aol.com
Adolescent asthma specialist

The Food Allergy Network
10400 Eaton Place, Suite 107
Fairfax, VA 22030
Tel: 703 691 3179; Fax: 703 691 2713
Toll-free: 1-800 929 4040
Email: fan@worldweb.net
Web: www.foodallergy.org

The Healthy House Institute
430 North Sewell Road
Bloomington, IN 47408
Tel: 812 332 5073
Web: www.hhinst.com
Publications and video tapes

US Consumer Product Safety Commission
Washington DC 20207
Toll-free: 1-800 638 2772
Email: info@cpsc.gov
Web: www.cpsc.gov

Equipment Manufacturers and Suppliers

A1 Vacuum & Allergy Control Specialists
78 Church Street
Saratoga Springs, NY 12866
Tel: 518 587 8263; Fax: 518 587 5792
Toll-free: 1-888 320 0004
Email: mail@a1allergy.com
Web: www.a1allergy.com
*Anti-mite bedding covers, anti-mite control
products, central and portable vacuum
cleaners, toys, washable bedding*

AFM Enterprises Inc
3251 Third Avenue
San Diego, CA 92103
Tel: 619 239 0321; Fax: 619 239 0565
Toll-free: 1-800 239 0321
Web: www.afmsafecoat.com
*Carpet care and cleaning products,
low-VOC paints and finishes, wood
and masonry sealers*

Allergy Control Products
96 Danbury Road
Ridgefield, CT 06877
Fax: 203 431 8963
Toll-free: 1-800 422 DUST
Web: www.allergycontrol.com
*Air cleaners, anti-mite bedding covers,
cleaning products, vacuum cleaners*

Allergy Home Care Products
(ComfortLiving.com)
630 East Diamond Avenue
Gaithersburg, MD 20877
Tel: 301 987 7787; Fax: 301 987 7975
Toll-free: 1-800 327 4382
Web: www.allergyhomecare.com
*Anti-mite powders and sprays,
dehumidifiers, face masks, high-filtration
vacuum cleaners, humidity gauge, mold-
resistant shower curtains*

Allergy Relief Shop Inc
3360 Andersonville Highway
Andersonville, TN 37705
Tel: 423 494 4100
Toll-free: 1-800 626 2810
Web: www.allergyreliefshop.com
Air filtration, cleaning products, consultancy service, cotton bedding, microbiology lab, paints, sealers, and solvents

Allergy Store
3504 South University Drive
Davie, FL 33328
Tel: 954 472 0128; Fax: 954 474 0133
Email: allergy@allergystore.com
Web: www.allergystore.com
Air filters, air-conditioning duct cleaning, anti-mite bedding products, cleaning products, dust mite control products, HEPA/ULPA vacuum cleaners, zeolite odor-control products

American Allergy Supply
PO Box 722022
Houston, TX 77272
Tel: 713 995 6110
Toll-free: 1-800 321 1096
Email: american@netropolis.net
Web: www.americanallergy.com
Air cleaners, anti-mite bedding covers, anti-mite sprays and powders, high filtration portable vacuum cleaners, mold inhibitor, nebulizers

Beam Industries
1700 West 2nd Street
PO Box 788
Webster City, IA 50595
Tel: 515 832 4620
Toll-free: 1-800 423 2682
Web: www.beamvac.com
Central vacuum systems

Bentley Mills
14641 East Don Julian Road
City of Industry, CA 91746
Toll-free: 1-800 423 4709
Low-emission carpets

California Closets
1000 Fourth Street, Suite 800
San Rafael, CA 94901
Tel: 415 256 8500; Fax: 415 256 8501
Toll-free: 1-800 873 4264
Web: www.calclosets.com
Custom-designed closet storage, including laminated-encased particleboard; in-home consultations

Chemical Specialties Inc
200 East Woodlawn Road, Suite 250
Charlotte, NC 28217
Tel: 704 522 0825
Toll-free: 1-800 421 8661
Wood treatments

Dwyer Products Corp
418 North Calumet Avenue
Michigan City, IN 46360
Tel: 219 874 5236
Toll-free: 1-800 441 1107
Web: www.dwyer.kitchens.com
Metal cabinetry

Easy Breathe Ltd
1781 Kingsdale Center, Suite 125
Columbus, OH 43221
Fax: 614 488 2000
Toll-free: 1-800 735 4772
Web: www.easybreathe.com
Allergy-friendly products, including anti-dust mite allergy sprays, anti-mite bedding protection, electrostatic dust cloths, electrostatic furnace filters, HEPA air cleaners, vent covering kits

Junckers Hardwood Inc
4920 East Landon Drive
Anaheim, CA 92807
Tel: 714 777 6430; Fax: 714 777 6436
Solid, prefinished hardwood flooring

Kitchens and Baths by Don Johnson
Suite 1375, Merchandise Mart
Chicago, IL 60654
Tel: 847 548 2436
Metal cabinets

Medite Corp
2685 North Pacific Highway
PO Box 4040
Medford, OR 97501
Tel: 541 773 2522
Toll-free: 1-800 676 3339
Web: www.sierrapine.com
Particleboard with no formaldehyde glue

Midwest Veneer & Pressing Inc
PO Box 572
5201 260th Street
Wyoming, MN 55092
Tel: 612 462 4389
Web: www.midwestveneer.com
Custom-veneered products

One Stop Allergy Shop
Web: stopallergy.com
Anti-dust mite powders and sprays, bedding, dehumidifiers, mite-detection kit, washable stuffed toys

Sebo America
6860 South Dallas Way
Englewood Village, CO 80112
Tel: 800 334 6614; Fax: 303 409 7786
Web: www.sebo-vacuums.com
High-filtration portable vacuum cleaners

Shaker Shops West
5 Inverness Way
PO Box 487
Inverness, CA 94937
Tel: 415 669 7256
Shaker-style solid wood furniture in kit form; overseas orders

State Allergy
3143 West Kennedy Blvd
Tampa, FL 33609
Tel: 813 872 7844; Fax: 813 874 8528
Toll-free: 1-888 841 4826
Web: www.stateallergy.com
Anti-dust mite powders, cleaning products, vacuum cleaners, vent covers

Therma-Stor (DEC International Inc)
1919 South Stoughton Road
PO Box 8050
Madison, WI 53708
Tel: 608 222 5301; Fax: 608 222 1447
Toll-free: 1-800 533 7533
Web: www.thermastor.com
Whole-house and single-room dehumidifiers and air-conditioning

Tucson Cooperative Warehouse
350 South Toole Avenue
Tucson, AZ 85701
Tel: 520 884 9951
Toll-free: 1-800 350 2667
Web: www.tcwfoodcoop.com
Organic 100 per cent cotton clothing, personal-care products

Venmar Ventilation Inc
550 Blvd Lemire
Drummondville, Quebec,
Canada J2C 7W9
Tel: 819 477 6226; Fax: 819 475 2660
Toll-free: 1-800 567 3855 (Canada
& USA)
Mechanical ventilation system

Wilsonart International
2400 Wilson Place
PO Box 6110
Temple, TX 76503
Tel: 254 207 7000
Toll-free: 1-800 433 3222
Website: www.wilsonart.com
Solid-surface countertops

Woodard & Greenstein
506 East 74th Street, 5th floor
New York, NY 10021
Tel: 212 794 9404
Toll-free: 1-800 332 7847
American country-style solid wood furniture,
cotton area rugs and stair runners

Wrisbo Co
5925 148th Street West
Apple Valley, MN 55124
Tel: 612 891 2000
Toll-free: 1-800 321 4739
Radiant floor heating

UNITED KINGDOM

Organizations

ASBA Architects Ltd
The Archway
373 Anlaby Road
Hull, Yorkshire HU3 6AB
Tel: 01482 576323; Fax: 01482 576325
Helpline: 0800 387310
Nationwide association of architects
specializing in domestic self-build,
refurbishment or extension projects

Anaphylaxis Campaign
PO Box 149
Fleet, Hants GU13 0FA
Tel: 01252 542029; Fax: 01252 377140
Web: www.anaphylaxis.org

British Allergy Foundation
Deepdene House
30 Bellegrove Road
Welling, Kent DA16 3BY
Tel: 020 8303 8525
Helpline: 020 8303 8583
Web: www.allergyfoundation.com
"Seal of approval" for allergy-related
products

Consumers Association (WHICH)
2 Marylebone Road
London NW1 4DX
Tel: 020 7830 8500; Fax: 020 7830 6220
Web: www.which.net

National Asthma Campaign
Providence House
Providence Place
London N1 0NT
Tel: 020 7226 2260; Fax: 020 7704 0740
Helpline: 0845 701 0203
Web: www.asthma.org.uk

National Asthma and Respiratory
   Training Centre for health professionals
The Athenaeum
10 Church Street
Warwick, Warks CV34 4AB
Tel: 01926 493313; Fax: 01926 493224
Email: enquiries@nartc.org.uk
Web: nartc.org.uk

National Eczema Society
163 Eversholt Street
London NW1 1BU
Tel: 020 7388 4097; Fax: 020 7388 5882
Helpline: 020 7388 3444
Web: www.eczema.org

UCB Institute of Allergy
UCB House
3 George Street
Watford, Herts WD1 8UH
Tel: 01923 211811; Fax: 01923 299002
Web: www.diseasemanagement.ucb.be
Allergy awareness publications & leaflets

Equipment Manufacturers
   ### and Suppliers

Advanced Allergy Technologies Ltd
187a Ashley Road
Hale, Cheshire WA15 9SQ
Tel: 0161 929 5549; Fax: 0161 929 6825
Email: allergy@allergy.uk.com
Web: allergy.uk.com
Anti-mite barrier covers and allergen
home analysis tests

Air Improvement Centre
23 Denbigh Street
London SW1V 2HF
Tel: 020 7834 2834; Fax: 020 7630 8485
Web: www.air-improvement.co.uk
Air conditioning units, air purifiers,
dehumidifiers, ionizers

Allerayde
3 Sanigar Court
Whittle Close, Newark
Notts NG24 2BW
Tel: 01636 613444; Fax: 01636 611186
Email: allerayde@aol.com
Anti-mite barrier covers, cleaning
powders and sprays for allergy control,
vacuum cleaners

Allergy Relief Products Ltd
Mansion House
Mansion Road
Southampton, Hants SO15 3BP
Tel: 023 8033 2919/8058 6709
Fax: 023 8933 2919/8067 6226
Anti-mite barrier bedding covers
and made-to-order barrier covers for
fabric-upholstered furniture

Atmospheric Solutions Ltd
Unit 23Y
Bond's Mill Estate
Bristol Road
Stonehouse, Glos GL10 3RF
Tel: 01453 825005
Order line: 0870 120 1262
Web: www.atmospherics.co.uk
Ozone eliminator

Baxi Ltd
20 Roman Way
Ribbleton
Preston, Lancs PR2 5BB
Tel: 01772 693 700; Fax: 01722 693701
Web: www.baxi.com
*Mechanical ventilation whole-house and
half-house system with heat recovery*

Boots Customer Services
Tel: 0845 0708090
Web: www.boots.co.uk
*Anti-mite bedding covers and sprays,
hypoallergenic and non-scented household
and cosmetic products, ionizers, smooth-
seamed baby clothing*

Chelmer Heating Services Ltd
Unit 4B, Baddow Park
West Hanning Field Road
Great Baddow
Chelmsford, Essex CM2 7SY
Tel: 01245 471111; Fax: 01245 471117
Email: chelmer@a1freenet.co.uk
*Condensing boilers, mechanical ventilation
system with heat recovery and comfort
cooling, underfloor heating*

Chris Drayson
The Gatehouse
Home Park Terrace
Hampton Court Road
Kingston, London KT1 4AE
Tel: 020 8943 0430
Interior design consultancy

Clement Clarke International Ltd
Airmed House
Edinburgh Way
Harlow, Essex CM20 2TT
Tel: 01279 414969; Fax: 01274 456304
Web: www.clement-clarke.com
Nebulizers, peak flow meters

David Robbens Underfloor Heating
    Systems Ltd
Unit 2, Old Forewood Lane
Crowhurst, East Sussex TN33 9AE
Tel: 01424 830140; Fax: 01424 830160
Email: robbens@underfloorheating.co.uk
Web: underfloorheating.co.uk
Underfloor central heating

Derwent Adept
134 Sheffield Road
Dronfield, Sheffield S18 2GE
Tel: 01246 292019; Fax: 01246 292012
Email: adept100@compuserve.com
Portable air cleaners, radiator dust filters

eco-co products (AF)
Birchwood
Briar Lane
Croydon, Surrey CR0 5AD
Tel: 020 8777 3121; Fax: 020 8777 3393
Web: www. ecozone.co.uk
*Chemical-free laundry balls which
replace soaps and detergents; other
environmentally friendly household
and personal care products*

Electrolux Floorcare
101 Oakley Road
Luton, Beds LU4 9QQ
Tel: 08706 055055; Fax: 01582 588380
Web: www.electrolux.com
High-filtration portable vacuum cleaners

FabDeck Ltd
Grange Road
Ellesmere, Shropshire, SY12 9DG
Tel: 01691 627200; Fax: 01691 627222
Email: sales@fabdeck.com
Web: www.darikool.demon.co.uk
*Whole-house dehumidifiers
(UK Therma-Stor distributors)*

Golden Key
1 Hare Street
Sheerness, Kent ME12 1AH
Tel: 01795 663403; Fax: 01795 661356
Email: golden_key@hotmail.com
Send SAE for product catalogue
Medical identification jewellery

Hampton Ventilation Ltd
Doveton House
129 Andover Road
Newbury, Berks RG14 6JJ
Tel: 01635 569933; Fax: 01635 40704
Email: john@fieldenj.freeserve.co.uk

Health Beds Ltd
Sarah Street
Rotherham, South Yorkshire S61 1EF
Tel: 01709 56193/559977
Low-allergen beds

Heat Profile
Internal Climate Control
Unit 1, Walnut Tree Park
Walnut Tree Close
Guildford, Surrey GU1 4TR
Tel: 01483 537000; Fax: 01483 537500
Email: contact@heatprofile.co.uk
Web: www.heatprofile.co.uk
Radiant skirting (base) board heating

Hoover European Appliance Group
Pentrebach
Merthyr Tydfil, CF48 4TU
Tel: 01685 721222; Fax: 01685 382946
High-filtration vacuum cleaners

IKEA
The Old Power Station
Valley Park
Purley Way
Croydon, CR0 4U2
Tel: 020 8208 5601
Web: www.ikea.com
*Streamlined, laminated-encased
board-based furniture, solid wood items,
bookcases and cabinets with glass doors,
sofas (couches) with washable covers*

Junckers
Wheaton Court Commercial Centre
Wheaton Road
Witham, Essex CM8 3UJ
Tel: 01376 517512; Fax: 01376 514401
Web: www.junckers.co.uk
Solid, prefinished hardwood flooring

Khars (UK) Ltd
Unit 2 West
68 Bognor Road
Chichester, West Sussex PO19 2NS
Tel: 01243 778747; Fax: 01243 531237
Web: www.khars.se
Solid, prefinished hardwood flooring

Kingsmead Carpets
Caponacre Industrial Estate
Cumnock, Ayrshire KA18 1SH
Tel: 01290 421511; Fax: 01290 424211
Web: www.kingsmead.carpetinfo.co.uk
Anti-allergy (anti-mite) carpets

Lakeland Paints
Unit 19, Lake District Business Park
Mint Bridge
Kendall, Cumbria LA9 6NH
Tel: 01539 732866
*Non-VOC, odourless, environmentally
friendly paints*

Richard Hudson and Sons Ltd (Medibed)
Dawson Court
Billington Road Industrial Estate
Burnley, Lancs BB11 5UB
Tel: 01282 430 224; Fax: 01282 439 306
Email: info@medibed.com
*Duvets and pillows, as well as protectors
for pillows, mattress, and duvets*

Medic-Alert Foundation
1 Bridge Wharf
156 Caledonian Road
London N1 9UU
Tel: 020 7833 3034; Fax: 020 7278 0647
Email: info@medicalert.co.uk
Medical identification jewellery

Medivac Healthcare Ltd
Wilmslow House
Grove Way
Wilmslow, Cheshire SK9 5AG
Tel: 01625 539401; Fax: 01625 539507
Web: www.medivac.co.uk
Air purifier, anti-mite barrier bedding covers, high-filtration vacuum cleaners, and dry-steam anti-mite process

Natural Collection
PO Box 2111
Bath BA1 2ZQ
Tel: 01225 442288; Fax: 01225 469673
Environmentally friendly products including unbleached, undyed cotton bedding

Nu-Heat
Unit 5, Lakes Court
Old Fore Street
Sidmouth, Devon EX10 8LP
Tel: 01395 578482; Fax: 01395 515502
Email: ufh@nu-heat.co.uk
Web: www.nu-heat.co.uk
Underfloor heating

Numatic International Ltd
Millfield Road
Chard, Somerset TA20 2GB
Tel: 01460 68480; Fax: 01460 269366
Web: www.numatic.co.uk
High-filtration vacuum cleaners

Rega Ubbink Ltd
Station Road
Sandy, Beds SG19 1BH
Tel: 01767 691291; Fax: 01767 692451
Email: mail@rega_uk.com
Humidity sensitive fans, mechanical ventilation system with heat recovery, passive stack ventilation

Sears, Roebuck & Co
33 Beverly Road
Hoffman Estates, ILL 60179
Tel: 847 286 2500
Web: www.sears.com
Allergy-related products, including air filters and air conditioning units

Sebo (UK) Ltd
The Merlin Centre
Cressex Business Park
High Wycombe, Bucks HP12 3QL
Tel: 01494 465533; Fax: 01494 461044
High-filtration vacuum cleaners

ServiceMASTER Ltd
ServiceMASTER House
Leicester Road
Anstey, Leics LE7 2AT
Tel: 0116 236 4646; Fax: 0116 236 2139
Carpet cleaning service, mite-killing and allergen-denaturing heat treatment for furniture, beds, soft toys, curtains (drapes)

Starkey Systems
St Martin's House
St Martin's Gate
Worcester, Worcs WR1 2DU
Tel: 01905 611041; Fax: 01905 27462
Email: beam@centralvacuums.co.uk
Web: www.centralvacuums.co.uk
Central vacuum cleaners

The Healthy House
Cold Harbour
Ruscombe
Stroud, GL6 6DA
Tel: 01453 752216; Fax: 01453 753533
Web: www.healthy-house.co.uk
Air purifiers, bedding barrier covers, allergen-friendly carpets, non-formaldehyde carpet underlay and adhesive, face masks, hand-held steam cleaner, non-VOC paint, and unbleached, undyed cotton bedding and clothing, including cotton sleepsuits and gloves

Talman Ltd (SOS Talisman)
21 Grays Corner
Ley Street
Ilford, Essex IG2 7RQ
Tel: 020 8554 5579; Fax: 020 8554 1090
Medical identification jewellery

Villavent Ltd
Avenue 2, Station Lane,
Industrial Estate
Witney, Oxon OX8 6YD
Tel: 01993 778481; Fax: 01993 779962
Central vacuum cleaner, mechanical ventilation with heat recovery

Vitalograph Ltd
Maids Moreton
Buckingham, Bucks MK18 1SW
Tel: 01280 827110; Fax: 01280 823302
Web: www.vitalograph.co.uk
Nebulizers, peak flow meters

Willan Building Services Ltd
2 Brooklands Road
Sale, Cheshire M33 3SS
Tel: 0161 962 7113; Fax: 0161 905 2085
Web: www.willan.co.uk
Passive ventilation system, wall and window trickle ventilators

Other Useful Addresses

ASH (Action on Smoking and Health)
102 Clifton Street
London EC2A 4HW
Tel: 020 7739 5902
Web: www.ash.org.uk
Information on tobacco; lobbying group and health charity for help in stopping smoking (see QUIT)

Asthma & Allergy Information
  & Research (AAIR)
Email: aair@globalnet.co.uk
Information on allergies, including house-dust mite sensitivity

Department of Health
Health and literature line: 0800 555 777
Publications and information on allergies and air pollution

Food Standards Agency
Ergon House
17 Smith Square
London SW1P 3JR
Consumer helpline: 0845 757 3012
Web: www.maff.gov.uk
Publications on food allergies and intolerance, food additives, labelling and safety, and nutrition

Health and Safety Executive
Information Centre
Broad Lane
Sheffield S3 7HQ
Tel: 0114 289 2345

QUIT
Victory House
170 Tottenham Court Road
London W1P 0HA
Tel: 020 7388 5775; Fax: 020 7388 5995
Quitline: 0800 00 22 00
Web: www.quit.org.uk
National charity helping smokers who want to stop smoking

Pollen count and air-pollution
  information
Daily Pollen Update
Tel: 0800 556 610
Pollen season only

Department of the Environment,
   Transport and Regions
Air pollution information: 0800 556 677
*Recorded message giving air-quality
information, including a forecast of pollution
levels*

Pollen Research Unit
Web: http//pollen.uk.worc.ac.uk
*General information on hayfever and
allergies, grass pollen monitoring, and useful
links across the world*

AUSTRALIA

Organizations

Asthma New South Wales
Unit 1/82-86 Pacific Highway
St Leonards, New South Wales 2065
Tel: 02 9906 3233; Fax: 02 9906 4493
Web: www.asthmansw.org.au

Asthma Northern Territory
Room 324, Block 4
Royal Darwin Hospital
Rocklands Drive
Tiwi, Northern Territory 0810
Tel: 8922 8817; Fax: 8922 8616
Email: athmant@mpx.com.au
Web: www.asthmaaustralia.org.au

Asthma Queensland
51 Ballow Street
Fortitude Valley
Queensland 4006
Tel: 07 3252 7677; Fax: 07 3257 1080
Web: www.asthma.org.au

Asthma South Australia
329 Payneham Road
Royston Park, South Australia 5070
Tel: 08 8362 6272; Fax: 08 8362 2818
Email: enquiry@asthmasa.org.au

Asthma Tasmania
Mailbox 5 McDougall Building
Ellerslie Road
Battery Point, Tasmania 7004
Tel: 03 6223 7725; Fax: 03 6224 2509
Email: asthmatas@bigpond.com.au
Web: www.asthmatas.org.au

Asthma Victoria
69 Flemington Road
North Melbourne, Victoria 3051
Tel: 03 9326 7088; Fax: 03 9326 7055
Email: afv@asthma.org.au
Web: www.asthma.org.au

Asthma Western Australia
36 Ord Street, West Perth 6005
Tel: 08 9481 1234; Fax: 08 9481 1292
Email: ask@asthmawa.org.au
Web: www.asthmawa.org.au

Australian Healthy Homes & Workplace
PO Box 734
Woodend, Victoria 3442
Tel: 03 5427 3175; Fax: 03 5427 3215
Email: bdesormeaux@healthyhouse.com
Web: www.healthyhouse.com
*Healthy house building consultancy
and central ventilation system*

Australian Healthy House Institute
PO Box 2155
Sunbury, Victoria 3429
Tel: 613 9740 3209; Fax: 613 9740 3099
Email: brandjes@ozonline.com.au
Web: www.envirobrokers.com.au
*Independent organization promoting
healthier indoor living and working
environments*

National Asthma Campaign (Australia)
1 Palmerston Crescent
South Melbourne, Victoria 3205
Tel: 03 9214 1476; Fax: 03 9214 1400
Email: nac@netlink.com.au

Equipment Manufacturers and Suppliers

Airflow Products Ltd
Rossmore House
123 Molesworth Street
Wellington, New Zealand
Tel: 04 499 1240; Fax: 04 499 1245
*Anti-mite barrier covers and allergen
home analysis tests*

Building Development Display Centre
332 Albert Street
East Melbourne, Victoria 3002
Tel: 03 9419 7488; Fax: 03 9417 2763
*Products suitable for low-allergen and
other building types on display*

Creative Wardrobe Company
4/3 Rhodes Street
West Ride, NSW 2114
Tel: 02 98 09 71 00; Fax: 02 98 08 50 94
*Custom-designed wardrobe storage and
cupboards, all made from laminated-
encased particleboard*

Dunlop Foam & Fibre Group
36 Commercial Drive
South Dandenong, Victoria 3175
Tel: 03 9215 2020; Fax: 03 9215 2010
Web: www.enduro.com.au
*Foam and polyester fibre fillings for
furniture and bedding; polyurethane
carpet underlay*

DuPont (Australia) Ltd
254 Canterbury Road
Bayswater, Victoria 3153
Tel: 03 9721 5900; Fax: 03 9721 5749
Web: www.dupont.com

Tilling Timber Pty Ltd
Orchard Street, Kilsyph, Victoria 3137
Tel: 03 9725 0222; Fax: 03 9725 3045
*Pre-finished solid timber flooring with
non-toxic coating*

Glossary

General terms

Adrenaline or epinephrine A natural hormone that is produced by the adrenal glands during exercise or while under stress, or frightened. It acts on the blood vessels to maintain blood pressure and circulation. Adrenaline (epinephrine) is administered by injection or by inhaler to treat the symptoms of a severe allergic reaction (anaphylaxis).

Aeroallergen Any allergen which is light enough to be carried in the air and inhaled, such as dander or pollen.

Allergen A foreign substance to which an individual becomes sensitized and against which the body's immune system produces a substance known as immunoglobulin E. An allergen may also be called an antigen.

Allergy Abnormal or inappropriate reaction of the body's immune system to a substance that would normally be harmless (allergen).

Allergic reactions A reaction of the body's immune system to an allergen, causing allergic symptoms.

Anaphylaxis A severe allergic reaction which can lead to collapse, even death.

Angioedema Swelling in the skin and underlying tissue.

Antibodies A protein produced in the body in response to an invading foreign material (known as an antigen), also called an "immunoglobulin".

Antigen Any foreign substance that provokes an immune response.

Antihistamine A drug that relieves the effects of histamine, a chemical produced by mast cells in the body during an allergic reaction. Histamine is one of several chemicals released by tissues when they are inflamed and causes many of the unpleasant symptoms that arise during inflammation.

Anti-inflammatory A medicine which reduces the swelling, redness, pain, and overheating in inflamed tissues of the body.

Atopy A hereditary tendency to develop a particular type of an allergic reaction (known as type 1 allergic reaction). The resulting allergic diseases include allergic rhinitis and eczema. About 40–50 per cent of the population are atopic, but people who are atopic do not necessarily have any symptoms.

Bronchodilators Drugs used to treat asthma that relax the smooth muscles in constricted airways and, therefore, widen the airways so that breathing is easier. They are often used in acute asthmatic attacks to relieve symptoms. They do not prevent attacks occurring.

Bronchi Small airways in the lungs.

Bronchospasm Sudden contraction of the bronchi (one of the signs of asthma).

Corticosteroids A group of hormones produced by the adrenal glands which are essential to many aspects of the way the body functions, including metabolism and resistance to stress; man-made corticosteroids are used as powerful anti-inflammatory drugs in a severe allergic reaction and are often used to prevent symptoms occurring.

Cromoglycate (sodium) A medicine used to prevent allergic symptoms.

Dander Small scales from animal skin, which act as an allergen in some people, producing an allergic reaction.

Desensitization see hyposensitization and immunotherapy.

Emollient A cream or ointment which is used to soften and soothe inflamed skin in eczema.

Histamine Chemical released by mast cells and basophils; responsible for the itching and swelling of hay fever and other allergies.

House-dust mite A minute, eight-legged arachnid found worldwide in household dust, soft furnishings, carpets, and bed linen; responsible for producing an allergic reaction in 85 per cent of cases of allergic asthma.

Hyposensitization see immunotherapy.

Hypersensitivity An over-reaction by the immune system to a foreign substance that would normally be ignored. It involves the excess production of immunoglobulin E antibody, beginning a process that ultimately results in allergic symptoms.

Hyposensitivity see immunotherapy.

Immunoglobulin E (IgE) IgE is a family of immunoglobulins (also known as antibodies). It is normally present only in tiny amounts in the blood. A type of white blood cell called the B lymphocyte produces immunoglobulins as part of the body's immune defence system. There are several different families of immunoglobulins, of which immunoglobulin E is one family. During an allergic reaction, B lymphocytes overproduce massive amounts of immunoglobulin E, a process that ultimately results in allergic symptoms.

Immune memory Ability of the body's immune system to retain information about foreign substances and to respond to their presence on a future occasion. Once an individual has become sensitized to a foreign substance, subsequent exposure to the substance will automatically trigger a reaction by the immune system, resulting in allergic symptoms.

Immunoglobulin see antibodies.

Immunotherapy Injections of gradually increasing amounts of an allergen known to trigger a patient's allergic response by which it is hoped to desensitize the patient so that they no longer show an allergic reaction to the allergen. Best tried where a person is only allergic to a single or just a few allergens.

Inflammation A collection of localized events, for example redness of the skin due to widening of the blood capillaries, accumulation of blood or fluid, which occur in reaction to the presence of certain agents, such as cat dander.

Mucus Liquid secretion produced by the mucous glands, such as those found in the respiratory tract. Excessive secretion of mucus during an attack of asthma forms in the airways, which may be coughed up later as tiny, lump-like "plugs" following the attack.

Patch test Skin test for diagnosing contact eczemas.

Pollen Male semen of plants.

Pollinosis An allergy to pollen ("hay fever").

Prick test Skin test used to search for an allergy.

Prostoglandins A naturally occurring group of chemicals, widely spread throughout the body and involved in many body functions. They constrict smooth muscle in an allergic reaction and are responsible for the narrowing of the airways that occurs in an acute asthma attack.

Pruritus Itching.

RAST A test for detecting IgE antibodies specifically involved in certain allergic reactions.

Rhinitis Inflammation of the membrane lining the nose (also known as the nasal mucosa), resulting in sneezing and congestion ("stuffiness") of the nasal passages or a runny nose. Seasonal rhinitis is popularly known as hay fever (pollinosis), while perennial rhinitis occurs all year around.

Sensitization This occurs when a person first encounters a substance which on subsequent exposures provokes an allergic reaction in the person. The substance is known as an allergen.

Theophylline A drug used to treat asthma, which has a bronchodilatory effect. *See also* bronchodilators.

Topical treatment This is applied directly on to the affected part of the body.

Vasoconstrictor A substance which constricts the tiny arteries – the arterioles – and can prevent or treat congestion as a result.

Building and home terms

Air conditioning Full air conditioning provides control over the temperature and humidity of air in a building. More commonly, temperature control only is provided to give comfort cooling in hot weather. Central system: the air conditioning unit distributes conditioned air throughout the building. Split system: a single outdoor unit connected to separate room units in each conditioned room. Portable or conditioning unit: provides local cooling. It requires a permanent or temporary duct connection to the outside to discharge the hot air produced.

Air filter Gaseous: a filter that can remove contaminated gases from air. Particulate: a filter that removes airborne particles from an air stream passing through it. HEPA (High Efficiency Particulate Air): a filter capable of removing particles below 1 micron in diameter.

Central heating Central heating provides a heat source, such as a boiler, a means of distributing the heat around the house, such as hot water pipes, and something to emit the heat into the room, such as a radiator.

Combustion by-products Burning any fossil fuel produces a mixture of combustion products, depending on the type of fuel and the efficiency of combustion. Some products are dangerous or even fatal, such as carbon monoxide produced by a poorly maintained gas burner.

Condensation The deposition of liquid water from moist air which is cooled below its dewpoint.

Cooker or range hood A hood mounted over a cooking hob which extracts the steam and fumes from cooking. The fumes are best discharged to the outside; in recirculating models, the fumes are passed through a carbon filter to remove odours and returned to the kitchen.

Dampness Unwanted or excessive moisture in a building. It may take the form of moisture condensing on a cold surface, or excessive moisture absorbed in the building structure.

Dehumidifier A device which removes moisture from the air. Most incorporate a small refrigeration unit which condenses water out of the air.

Dewpoint The temperature at which a volume of air becomes saturated when cooled. Further cooling results in condensation. Energy efficiency (or energy conservation): the reduction of fuel and energy consumption in the home by a combination of insulation, efficient appliances, and controlled use.

Draught-proofing (weather-stripping) Draught-proofing a house reduces unwanted ventilation, giving more comfort and lower bills. Attention should be paid to all routes of air leakage, such as skirting (base) boards, floorboards, and any air holes in the walls or ceiling for pipework.

Extractor (exhaust) fan A fan that draws air from a room and discharges it to the outside.

Forced air heating Air is heated by a central source and distributed throughout the house using ducts. Warm air is transferred into rooms via registers and eventually returns to the heat source for recirculation.

Formaldehyde A pungent, irritant gas which is a health hazard in high concentrations. It is used in the production of some resin glues and insulation materials, which are found in most homes.

Flue Open: An open-flue combustion appliance draws in room air to provide the oxygen needed for combustion and provision must be made for this air supply by ensuring permanent ventilation. The combustion products are discharged to the outside through a flue. Closed: also known as a room-sealed appliance. The combustion air is drawn from the outside; the outdoor terminal incorporates both air intake and flue gas exhaust. Some appliances use a small fan to ensure satisfactory discharge of the flue gases.

Healthy housing Housing that provides a safe and healthy environment for its inhabitants. A wider definition includes good mental health and social well-being in addition to physical health and safety.

Humidity A measure of the amount of water vapour held in the air. Absolute: the quantity of water vapour contained in a cubic meter of air. It is measured in grams of water per kilogram of air. Relative (RH): the humidity of a volume of air, expressed as a percentage of the amount of water vapour the air could contain if saturated. The RH depends on both the absolute humidity and the temperature of the air in question. Saturated air: air which contains as much water vapour as it can hold and which has by definition a relative humidity of 100 per cent.

Humidifier A device which adds water vapour to the air, either in the form of steam or fine droplets of water.

Ionizer A device which imparts an electrostatic charge to the air molecules, which are then termed ions. The ions encourage any dust particles in the air to stick to surfaces, such as walls, and so the ionizer acts to clean the air. Benefits to mood and breathing have been claimed.

Insulation Thermal insulation in a house reduces the heat loss in winter. This results in more comfort, lower heating bills, and warmer surfaces, which in turn reduces condensation and mould growth.

Mechanical ventilation Ventilation driven by mechanical means, such as an electric fan. Balanced: mechanical ventilation system where both the intake of outside air and the exhaust of inside air are powered by fans. Balanced ventilation units may serve a single room or a whole house. Half-house: a balanced mechanical ventilation system installed in the loft of a house and serving upstairs rooms only, and normally complemented by a kitchen extract ventilator. Whole-house: a balanced mechanical ventilation system serving the whole house, usually incorporating filtration of incoming air and heat recovery. With heat recovery: a mechanical ventilation system where energy is recovered from the outgoing air and transferred to the incoming air. With energy recovery: a mechanical

ventilation system where energy is recovered from the outgoing air and transferred to the incoming air. Usually the same as heat recovery. With desiccant wheel: a device that exchanges both heat and moisture between the two airstreams of inside air and outside air. It can recover energy in a whole-house ventilation system, whether the house is being heated or cooled, humidified or dehumidified, and so has application in a wide range of climates.

Natural ventilation Ventilation that takes place by the natural forces of wind and temperature; examples are open windows, chimneys, and passive-stack ventilation. Passive-stack ventilation: a natural ventilation system consisting of extract ducts running from the kitchen, bathroom, and laundry up to the roof, together with air inlets in habitable rooms. Some degree of control is possible using dampers which respond to changes in humidity.

Solvent A liquid used to dissolve other substances, such as white spirit (mineral spirit) or carbon tetrachloride. Solvents are a source of VOCs (see below).

Trickle ventilator A ventilator designed to provide background ventilation. Trickle ventilators usually incorporate a grille to guard against weather and flies, and are commonly fitted in a window frame.

Ventilation The replacement of stale air in a building by air from outside.

Volatile Organic Compound (VOCs) This term covers the wide range of vapours given off by organic compounds, such as plastics or glues. Identifying the large number of individual compounds is a complex task, and it is conventional to lump them together as VOC concentration, to give a general measure of air quality.

Water vapour Water that exists as an invisible gas in the air. Cooking, drying clothes, and human sweating and breathing all put water vapour into the air.

Bibliography

DISEASE-RELATED

There are many books on allergies written with the layperson in mind. The following is a recently published selection of these.

Allergies in general

Clough, Joanne, *Allergies at Your Fingertips*, Class Publishing, London, 1997

Davies, Professor Robert, *Understanding Allergies and Hayfever*, Family Doctor Publications and British Medical Association, London, 1995

Rothera, Ellen, *Perhaps it's an Allergy*, Foulsham, Chippenham, 1998

Anaphylaxis

Williams, Dr Deryk, Williams, Anna, and Croker, Laura, *Life-threatening Allergic Reactions*, Piatkus Books, London, 1997

Asthma

Levy, Mark, Hilton, Sean, and Barnes, Greta, *Asthma at Your Fingertips: The Comprehensive Asthma Reference Book for the 1990s*, Class Publishing, London, 1997 (2nd edition)

Lewis, Jenny (with National Asthma Campaign), *The Asthma Handbook*, Vermilion, London, 1996

Youngson, R. M., *Living with Asthma*, Sheldon Press, London, 1995

Eczema

Atherton, Dr David J., *Eczema in Childhood: The Facts*, Oxford University Press, Oxford, 1995 (revised edition)

Lewis, Jenny (with National Eczema Society), *The Eczema Handbook: A Guide to the Causes, Symptoms and Treatments*, Vermilion, London, 1994

Youngson, R. M., *Coping With Eczema*, Sheldon Press, London, 1995

Hayfever

Brostoff, Dr Jonathan and Gamlin, Linda, *Hayfever: How to Cope With Hayfever, Asthma and Related Problems*, Bloomsbury Publishing, London, 1997 (3rd edition)

OTHER THERAPIES

Many people turn to non-orthodox therapies in their search for relief from allergy symptoms. The following book gives a sensible outline of the different therapies on offer without raising impossible hopes.

Rowlands, Barbara and Watkins, Dr Alan, *Alternative Answers to Asthma and Allergies*, Marshall Publishing, London, 1999

STRESS MANAGEMENT

Stress is not a cause of allergy but it can make symptoms worse. Practising stress avoidance and learning to manage stress may help some people to alleviate their allergic symptoms.

Brewer, Dr Sarah, *Good Housekeeping's The Ultimate Stress Buster*, Ebury Press, London, 1999

Patel, Dr Chandra, *The Complete Guide to Stress Management*, Vermilion, London, 1996 (revised edition)

HOUSE CONSTRUCTION AND DESIGN

The following titles are just a few of the increasing number being published on building healthy homes. Many of them are written with the chemically sensitive person in mind, but they also contain much background information on indoor pollutants and the systems involved in a house, such as ventilation and heating.

Baker, Paula, Elliott, Erica, and Banta, John, *Prescriptions for a Healthy House: A Practical Guide for Architects, Builders and Homeowners*, Inwood Press, Santa Fe, 1998

Bower, John, *Healthy House Building: A Design and Construction Guide*, The Healthy House Institute, Bloomington, 1997 (2nd edition)

Bower, John, *The Healthy House: How to Buy One, How to Build One, How to Cure One*, The Healthy House Institute, Bloomington, 1997 (3rd edition)

Bower, Lynn Marie, *The Healthy Household*, The Healthy House Institute, Bloomington, 1995

Huntington, Lucy, *Creating a Low-Allergen Garden*, Mitchell Beazley, London, 1998

Kruger, Anna, *H is for ecoHome*, Gaia Books Ltd, 1991

HOUSEHOLD CLEANING

The following is a well-researched, practical book that explains how to use everyday ingredients to clean your home effectively. It provides real alternatives to chemically laden, proprietary branded products.

Berthold-Bond, Annie, *Clean & Green or "458 Ways to Clean, Polish, Disinfect, Deodorize, Launder, Remove Stains – Even Wax Your Car Without Harming Yourself or the Environment"**, CERES Press, Woodstock, 1994

*Included by kind permission of CERES Press, PO Box 87, Woodstock, NY 12498, USA/email www.healthiest.diet.com. Paperback/softcover US$8.95 + $4.00 (surface mail)/$12.50 (air mail)

Index

Page numbers in *italic* refer to the illustrations

acaricides, 70, 82, 83
acid aerosols, 32
adhesives, 68
adrenaline, 47
aerosols, 69, 76
air conditioning, 43, 50, 58, 59, 121–3, 125
air fresheners, 69, *101*, 112
air grilles, 54, 55
air pollution: external, 32–3, *32–3*
    filters, 57, 58
    household air pollution, 34–5
    interior air quality, 50–9
airborne allergies, 14–17, *14*
airways, allergic reactions, *12*
allergen, definition, 13
allergic contact dermatitis, 18–19
allergies: airborne allergies, 14–17, *14*
    allergic reactions, 12–13
    contact allergies, 18–19
    contributory factors, 24
    definition, 13
    diagnosis, 44–5, *44*
    ingested (food) allergies, 20–1
    management, 44–7
Allergy House, Helsinki, 115
Alternaria, 43
alveolitis, allergic, 17
American Lung Association (ALA), 115,
    116, 118
anaphylaxis, 22–3, 47
animals, *15*, 24, 40–1, 50, 86, 90, 99
antihistamine, 45–6
anti-inflammatory therapy, 46–7
antileukotrienes, 46
architects, 116
art and hobby materials, 69
arthralgia, and food allergy, 20
Aspergillus, 42, 43
asthma, 14–15
    and air pollution, 33
    allergic reactions, *12*
    anti-inflammatory therapy, 46
    antileukotrienes, 46
    Asthma Victoria Breathe Easy campaign,
        115, 116, 124–5, *124–5*, 126

brittle asthma, 23
    exercise and, 27
    and food allergy, 20
    humidifiers, 59
    passive smoking and, 35
    peak-flow meters, *46*
    pet allergy, 40
    prevalence, 27
    reliever therapy, 47, *47*
    thunderstorm asthma, 30, 31
atopic eczema, 21
atopy, 13
attic conversions, 106, *106–7*
Australia, 115, 118–27
Australian Healthy House Institute,
    118
auto travel *see* car travel
avoiding allergens, 45

backing, carpet, 63
balanced-flue boilers, 109
barrier covers, bedding, 81, 82, *82*, 83,
    88, 89, 99
basement conversions, 106, 108–9, *108*
bath oils, 103
bathrooms, 53, 54, 55, 100–3, *100–3*
baths, *100*
bed linen, 76, 83, 88
bedding, 69, *80*, 82–3, *87*
bedrooms, 53, 54, 80–3, *80–3*
beds, 80, *81*, 82–3, *87*, 88
bedspreads, 83, 88
bee stings, 22, 112
benzyl benzoate, 76, 83, 89
biological washing products, 76–7
birch pollen, *15*, 20, *28*
birds, 41
blankets, 83
blinds, 65, 81
blood tests, 44–5
boilers, 55, 61, 109
bookshelves, *104*
Brandjes, Jon, 118
breathing, *14*
brittle asthma, 23
budgerigars, 41
building low-allergen houses, 116
bunk beds, 88

Canada, 118
car travel, 112
carbon monoxide, 32, 55, 61
carpets, 42–3, 62–3, 69, 74, 81, 92–3
case histories, 115
cats, 40, *40*, 50, 99
central heating, 55, 58–9, 60–1
ceramic tiled floors, 63, 64
chairs, office, *104*
charcoal air filters, 57
chemicals: allergic contact dermatitis,
    18–19, *18*
    contact urticaria, 19
    fly-killers, 98
    fragrances, 103
    garden chemicals, *111*
    household air pollution, 34–5
    interior air quality, 50
    VOCs, 68–9
children's play areas, 110
children's rooms, 86–9, *86–9*
chimneys, 61
Cladosporium, 43
cleaning houses, 72–3
    see also individual rooms
cleaning products, 68, 76–7, 92, 93, 99
clothes, 84–5
    children's, 87
    dry-cleaning, 69, 85
    easy-care, 69
    washing, 76–7, *84*, 85
clutter, dust and, 72
cockroaches, 24, 38–9, *38*, 94, 99, 100
coeliac disease, 21
combustion sources and by-products,
    60, 61
compost, *110*
condensation, 52, *52*, 53
conjunctivitis, 14, 16–17
    and air pollution, 33
    antihistamine, 46
    anti-inflammatory therapy, 46
    pet allergy, 40
conservatories, 24, *111*
contact allergies, 18–19
contact dermatitis, 76, 77, 103
contact urticaria, 18, 19
convection heating, 61

conversions, 106–9, *106–9*
cookers, 60, 61, 94, *95*, 96–7, 125
cooking methods, 96–7
cooktops *see* hobs
cork floors, 63
corticosteroids, 46
cosmetics, 102–3
cots, 89
cotton, 63, 84–5
cows, 41
curtains, 65, 81, *101*
cushions, *91*
cyclonic vacuum cleaners, 75

dairy products, 21
dampness, 24, 42, 53, 108
dehumidifiers, 58, 106, 108
denaturing agents, 70, 71
dermatitis, 18, 76, 103
Desmoreaux, Bernard, 118
detergents, 77
diagnosis, 44–5, *44*
diaper rash, *88*
digestive system, coeliac disease, 21
dock weed pollen, 29
dogs, 40–1, *41*, 99
doors, 123
double-glazing, 50, 52, 65
drainpipes, 109
drapes *see* curtains
draught-proofing, 50, 53, 56, 60, 113
drug treatment, 45–7
dry-cleaning, 69, 85, 93
dry steam cleaning, 70, 93
ducted cooker hoods, 97
ducts, *107*
dust, 72, 106, 125
    see also house-dust mites
duvets, 80, 81, 83, 88
dyes, 18

Eastern Energy, 124
eczema, 18–19
    anti-inflammatory therapy, 46
    atopic eczema, 21
    cleaning products and, 76, 77
    and food allergy, 20
    prevalence, 27
    skin care, 103
    soft-water and, 99
eggs, 21
electric blankets, 80
electrical equipment, home offices,
    104, *105*

electrostatic air filters, 57
emollients, 103
enzymes, biological washing products,
    76–7
exhaust fans *see* extractor fans
exercise, 27, 33, 126
extractor fans, 54, 55, 113
eyes *see* conjunctivitis

fabric conditioners, 77, 85, 99
fabrics, clothes, 84–5
family factors, 26–7
fig, weeping, 23
filters: air filters, 57, 58
    in cars, 112
    vacuum cleaners, 74–5
Finnish Allergy and Asthma Federation,
    115
Finnish Pulmonary Association, 115
fires, 60, 61, *91*
fish: food intolerance, 20
    pet allergies, 41
floors, 62–4, *63*, 69, *110*
    Asthma Victoria Breathe Easy
        campaign, 124–5
    basements, 109
    bathrooms, 100, *100*
    bedrooms, 81
    children's rooms, *86*
    conversions, *107*
    home offices, *104*
    kitchens, 94, *94*
    living rooms, 90, *91*, 92
    Sunbury Healthy House, 120–1
flowers, 24
    see also pollen
fly-killers, 98–9
food: anaphylaxis, 22–3
    additives, 20, 27
    allergies, 20–1, 45
    intolerance, 20
formaldehyde, 34, 69
    carpet backing, 63
    fabric treatments, 85
    in furniture, 68, 71, 92
    in insulation, 68, 109
    interior air quality, 50
    in paints, 68
    wall panelling, 65
fossil fuels, 32
fragrances, 103
freezers, *94*, 98
freezing bed linen, 83
friends, visiting, 113

fruit, 77, 98
fungi *see* mould spores
furniture, 70–1, *70–1*
    bedrooms, *80*
    children's rooms, *86*
    formaldehyde in, 68, 71, 92
    garden rooms, *111*
    home offices, *105*
    kitchens, *95*, 98, *98*
    living rooms, *90*, 92
    Sunbury Healthy House, 120

garages, 112–13
gardens, 110, *110–11*, 125
gas boilers, 109
gas convector heaters, 61
gas cookers, 34, 60, 61, 94, 96
gender differences, 27
gloves, 76
glue, formaldehyde, 71
gluten, coeliac disease, 21
grass pollens, 28–9, *29*, 30, *30*
grouting, tiled floors, 64
gutters, 109

hair products, 102
hand care, 77
hard-surface flooring, 63–4, *63*, 81, 92
hardwood floors, 64
hay fever, 15
    antihistamine, 45–6
    diagnosis, 45
    grass pollens, 29
    prevalence, 27
    thunderstorm asthma, 30
heat exchangers, 57
heat treatment, furnishings, 71
heating systems, 55, 60–1
    Asthma Victoria Breathe Easy
        campaign, 125
    bedrooms, 81
    conversions, *107*
    home offices, *105*
    humidifiers, 58–9
    living rooms, *91*
    Sunbury Healthy House, 123
hedges, *111*
HEPA air filters, 57, 58
HEPA-filter vacuum cleaners, 74–5
herbs, deterring flies, 98–9
histamine, 20, 46
hives, 19
hobby materials, 69
hobs, 96

holidays, 113
Holland, 115
home offices, 104–5, *104–5*
hoods, extractor, 55, *55*, 97
horses, 41
house-dust mites, 24, 36–7, *36*
   air-filtering units, 58
   in beds, 80, 82–3
   in carpets, 62
   in children's rooms, 86
   diagnosis of allergy, 44
   dogs and, 99
   dust and, 72
   in furnishings and fixtures, 70–1
   in home offices, 104
   and humidity, 52, 53
   in living rooms, 92
   in rugs, 63
   temperature and, 60
   and ventilation, 54
   washing clothes, 76
house plants, 59
household air pollution, 34–5
humidifiers, 58–9
humidity: bedrooms, 81
   dehumidifiers, 58, 106, 108
   house-dust mites and, 37
   interior air quality, 50, 52–3
   mould spores, 42
hygiene products, 69
hypersensitivity, 13
hypoallergenic, definition, 102

immune system, 26
   allergic reactions, 12–13
immunity, definition, 13
immunoglobulin E (IgE), 13, 44
immunotherapy, 47
inflammation, 13
ingested (food) allergies, 20–1
inhalers, 47, *47*
insects: cockroaches, 24, 38–9, *38*, 94,
      99, 100
   stings, 22, *22*, 112
   see also house-dust mites
insulation, 53, 60
   Asthma Victoria Breathe Easy
      campaign, 125
   in attics or basements, 109
   conversions, *106*
   interior air quality, 50, 52
   Sunbury Healthy House, 123
   urea-formaldehyde foam, 68, 109
interior air quality, 50–9

ionizers, 58
irritant dermatitis, 18–19, 76, 102

jewellery, medical-alert, 23

kitchens, 94–9, *94–9*
   ventilation, 53, 54, 55, *55*, 94, 97

labels, terminology, 102
lactase, 20
lampshades, *87*
lanolin, 84
latex allergy, 19, 22, 23, 76
laundry, 76–7, 85, 109
lawns, *110*
leather upholstery, 70
leukotrienes, 46
lifestyle factors, 27
lighting, 95, *107*
lime-based paints, 67
linoleum, 63, 64
living rooms, 90–3, *90–3*
loft conversions *see* attic conversions
lungs, *12*, *14*, 17

mast cells, 44
matting, 63
mattresses, 80, 81, *81*, 82–3, 88, 89
mechanical ventilation systems, 54, 121
mechanical ventilation with heat
      recovery (MVHR), 56–7
medical-alert jewellery, 23
medicine cabinets, *100*
medium-density fibreboard (MDF),
      71, 92
Melbourne, 115, 116, 118
metals, allergic contact dermatitis, 18
midges, 112
milk allergy, 20
mites, house-dust *see* house-dust mites
moisture barriers, 123
mosquitoes, 112
mothproofing agents, 85
mould spores, 24, 42–3, *42*
   avoiding, 42, 99, 113
   in basements, 108
   in carpets, 62
   and humidity, 52, *52*
   in wallpaper, 65

nettle rash, 19
neutrophil white cells, 13
nickel, 18
nitrogen dioxide, 32, 33, *33*, 34

nitrogen oxides, 60–1
nitrogen treatments, furnishings, 71
nose: airborne allergies, 14
   breathing through, *14*, 33
   rhinitis, 16
nut allergy, 20, 21, 22–3

offices, home, 104–5, *104–5*
oil paints, 66, 67
oral allergy syndrome, 20
ovens, cleaning, 96
oxygen, allergic alveolitis, 17
ozone, 32, 33, 58, 104

paints, *34*, 35, *35*, 65, 66–7, *66*, 68
panelled walls, 65
particulate matter, 32
passive smoking, 35, 61
passive stack ventilation, 53, 57
patch tests, *44*, 45
peanut allergy, 20, 22–3
Penicillium, 42, 43
perennial allergic conjunctivitis, 16–17
pets, *15*, 24, 40–1, 50, 86, 90, 99
pillows, 80, 81, 82, 83, 88, 91
Pirquet, Clemens Freiherr von, 12
plants, 111, *111*, *112*, 125
   allergic contact dermatitis, *19*, 19
   contact urticaria, 19
   cut flowers, 24
   house plants, 59
   and latex allergy, 23
   see also pollen
plaster, drying, 106
play areas, *110*
poison ivy, 19
poison oak, 19
poison sumak, 19
polishes, 77
pollen, 24, 28–31, *28–30*
   avoiding, 113
   conjunctivitis, 16
   cut flowers, 24
   hay fever, 15
   oral allergy syndrome, 20
pollution: air-filtering units, 58
   external air pollution, 32–3, *32–3*
   household air pollution, 34–5
   interior air quality, 50
   in kitchens, 96
   road-traffic, *17*, 32–3, *33*
   thunderstorm asthma, 30
polyester, 85
porches, *111*

portable heaters, 61
preservatives, 20, 103
pressure cookers, 96–7
primulas, 19, *19*
proteins: allergic reactions, 12–13
    protein-based paints, 67

quilts, 83, 88

radiant heating, 61
radiant skirting boards, 61
radiators, 61
ragweed pollen, 20, 29–30, *30*
refrigerators, *94*, 98
reliever therapy, 47
resin-based paints, 67
rhinitis, *13*, 14, 16
    and air pollution, 33
    antihistamine, 46
    anti-inflammatory therapy, 46
    and food allergy, 20
    pet allergy, 40
rings, 77
road-traffic pollution, *17*, 32–3, *33*
rodents, 41
roofs, *106*, 109
Rotterdam, 115
rugs, 63, 81, 92

scombroid poisoning, 20
seasonal allergic conjunctivitis, 16
secondary-glazing *see* double-glazing
Shades *see* blinds
shampoos, 102
sheds, 112–13, *113*
shower curtains, *101*
showers, *43*, 100, *101*
sinks, *95*
skin: allergic reactions, 12–13
    atopic eczema, 21
    contact allergies, 18–19, 103
    gardening and, 111
    irritant reactions, 102
    patch tests, *44*, 45
    skin care, 103
    skin-prick tests, 44, *44*, 45
skin scales, in dust, 72
smog, 32, *32*
smoking, 35, 61, 125
soaps, 103
soft furnishings, 70, 93, *107*
solvents, 66, 69, 76, 77, 93
spores *see* mould spores
stack ventilation, 53, 57

stain removers, 77, 85
steam cleaning, 70, 93
steroids, 46, 126
stings, 22, *22*, 112
stir-frying, 97
stone paint, 67
storage, in attics or basements, 109, *109*
stoves *see* cookers
studies, 104–5, *104–5*
sulphur dioxide, 32, 33, 34, 50, 60
Sunbury Healthy House, Melbourne,
    115, 116, 118–23, *118–23*

tannic acid, 70, 71
temperature, house-dust mites and, 37
terminology, 13
tests, diagnosis of allergy, 44–5, *44*
theophylline, 47
thunderstorm asthma, 30, 31
tiled floors, 63, 64
timber, conversions, *106*
tobacco smoke, 35, 61, 125
toiletries, 102–3
toilets, *100*
towels, *101*
toys, *86*, 89, *89*
traps, cockroach, 39
treatment of allergies, 45–7
tree pollens, 28, *28*, *30*
trickle ventilators, 54, 55, 65
trigger factors: asthma, 15
    outside the home, 112–13
tumble driers, 109
tyramine, 20

underfloor heating, *60*, 61
United States of America, 115
upholstery, 70
urea-formaldehyde foam insulation
    (UFFI), 68, 109
urticaria, 18, 19, 20, 46
utility rooms, *108*, 109

vacations, 113
vacuum cleaners, 63, 70–1, 74–5,
    74–5, 125
vapour barriers, 123
varnishes, 66, 68
vegetables, 77, 98
ventilation, 50, 52
    Asthma Victoria Breathe Easy
        campaign, 124
    bathrooms, 100
    improving, 54–5

ventilation (cont.)
    kitchens, 53, 54, 55, *55*, 94, 97
    natural ventilation, 53
    Sunbury Healthy House, 121
    ventilation systems, 56–7
vents, *107*
vernal keratoconjunctivitis, 17
vinyl flooring, 63, 64
vinyl upholstery, 70
volatile organic compounds (VOCs),
    34–5, 50, 66, 68–9, 120

wall coverings, 64–5
wallpaper, 64–5, *65*
walls: bathrooms, *101*
    bedrooms, *81*
    children's rooms, *87*
    home offices, *104*
    kitchens, *94*
    living rooms, *91*
washing: carpets, 92
    clothes, 76–7, *84*, 85
    hands, 77
washing machines, 108, 109
washing powders, 76–7, 99
wasp stings, 22, *22*, 112
water-based paints, 66
water-filter vacuum cleaners, 75
water softeners, 99
water vapour: in bathrooms, 100
    humidity, 50, 52–3
    in kitchens, 94
weather, 30–1, 32
weather stripping *see* draught-proofing
weed pollens, 29–30, *30*
white blood cells, 13
windows, 65
    bathrooms, *101*
    bedrooms, *81*
    children's rooms, *86*
    conversions, *107*
    home offices, *105*
    kitchens, *94*
    living rooms, *91*
    Sunbury Healthy House, 123
    trickle ventilators, 54, 55, 65
Wood, Leisl, 115, 116, 125–7
wood preservatives, 67, 68
wooden floors, *63*, 64, 92
wooden furniture, *70*, 71
wooden panelling, 65
wool, 63, 84
workshops, 113
worktops, *95*, 98

Acknowledgments

Photographic acknowledgments in source order

Abode/Ian Parry 113/Spike Powell 25; Allerayde 82; Allergy and Asthma Federation, Finland 114; Heather Angel 28, 29 top right; The Asthma Foundation of Victoria/BREATHE EASY TM/Eastern Energy 124, 125, 126, 127; Bubbles/David Robinson 40; Camera Press Ltd 112; Environmental Images/Martin Bond 17/Vanessa Miles 33; Elizabeth Whiting Associates 108; Garden Picture Library/Steven Wooster 59; Habitat UK 49 (inset); Home Beautiful/Sunbury Healthy House 118–119, 120, 121, 122–123; Houses & Interiors/Verne 2, 92; IKEA 89; Images Colour Library 26, 88; The Interior Archive/Fritz von der Schulenburg 80–81/Andrew Wood 94–95; International Interiors/Paul Ryan 106–107/Frances Halliday 110–111; IPC/Homes and Gardens/Hannah Lewis 70/Pia Tryde 93/ Living Etc/Peter Aprahamian 15, 55; Junckers Solid Hardwood Flooring 63, 73; Kahrs 78, 97; Miele Company Ltd 96; Octopus Publishing Group Ltd 19, /Dominic Blackmore 6, 100–101, 104–105, 109, 129/Tim Clinch 51/Jeremey Hopley 84/James Johnson 20/James Merrell 34, 62, 86–87, /Kevin Summers 24/Simon Upton 64, 71, 83, 90–91, 98; Mountain Breeze (0161 947 3000) 58; N.H.P.A./Stephen Dalton 38; Rehau 60; Science Photo Library 52/Dr Jeremy Burgess 22/Mark Clarke 46/Ralph Eagle 30 bottom left/Eye of Science 36, 42/Keith Kent 31/James King-Holmes 44 bottom right/John Mead 32/Saturn Still 44 bottom centre/Andrew Syred 29 top centre; SEBO (UK) LTD 75; Starkey Systems 74; Tony Stone Images 21, 30 bottom centre, 35, 66, 103/Doug Armand 37/Christopher Bissell 65/Christoph Burki 4–5/Roger Charity 18/Donna Day 41/Mark Douet 13/Dale Durfee 43/Alain le Garsmeur 10–11, 48–49, 128–129/Claude Guillaumin 102/Walter Hodges 117/S Lowry/Univ. Ulster 1/John Millar 47, 77/Andreas Pollok 11/Jon Riley 16/Camille Tokerud 27

Acknowledgments

Our thanks go especially to: Mrs Carol Martin for her unfailing secretarial support and assistance; Dr Donald McIntyre, ventilation expert, Indoor Climate Services, Chester, UK, and Dr Colin Hunter of the Building Research Establishment, Watford, UK, for their invaluable advice and assistance in preparing the manuscript for this book; Carin Lavery of Asthma Foundation Victoria, Australia, Leisl Wood of Mansfield, Victoria, Australia, Bernard Desmoreaux and Jan Brandjes of the Australian Healthy House Institute, Sunbury, Victoria, Australia, and Susanna Palkonen of the Finnish Allergy and Asthma Federation, Helsinki, Finland, for their time and help in preparing the case histories; Marsha Williams and the press office of the National Asthma Campaign, London, UK, for their patient assistance.

We would also like to thank the following people for their time and advice in compiling this book: Eleanor Brown, librarian, Electricity Association Technology Ltd, Chester, UK; Craig Butler, Derwent Adept; Dr Derrick Crump of the Building Research Establishment, Watford, UK; Chris Drayson, interior designer of the National Asthma Campaign's low-allergen home, Milton Keynes, UK; Victoria Flint, Publications, National Asthma Campaign, London, UK; John Hardy, architect of Hardy Associates, Bristol, UK; Howard Kloester of Hurricane Advertising and Marketing, Fitzroy, Victoria, Australia; Sonja Jeltes, Netherlands Asthma Foundation, Leusden; Claire Marris for her insight into building a low-allergen home and caring for a child with allergies; Martine Packer of Packer Forbes Communications, London, UK; Carol Peek, British Allergy Foundation, Welling, UK; Richard Porteous and Jonathan Starkey, directors, Starkey Systems, Worcester, UK; Don Pringle, Servicemaster, Dublin, Eire; Mike Rhodes, director, Allerayde, Newark, UK; Maxima Skelton, director, The Healthy House, Stroud, UK; Colin Taylor, managing director, Medivac, Wilmslow, UK; and Josine van den Bogaard, The GGD Rotterdam, Netherlands.

Our grateful thanks also go to the following for permission to incorporate material from their publications: Ceres Press (Woodstock, NY, USA), publisher, and Annie Berthold-Bond, author, for cleaning recipes 50–3 (see p. 101), recipe 84 (see p. 76), recipes 177 and 181 (see p. 101) from *Clean & Green*; John Fielden of Hampton Ventilation Ltd, Newbury, UK (see p. 54, table); Mitchell Beazley (London, UK), publisher, and Lucy Huntington, author, of *Creating a Low-Allergen Garden* (see pp. 110–113); National Eczema Society, London, UK; Des Whitrow, author of *House Dust Mites: How They Affect Asthma, Eczema and Other Allergies*; Dr Ian White, author of an article on cosmetics and allergens published in issue 1 of the British Allergy Foundation's *Allergy Free* magazine (see pp. 102–103); Ian West, director, Lakeland Paints, Kendall, UK (see p. 67, table).

Thank you also to the following people for their input and support during the writing of this book: Philip Arrand, Annie and Lawrence Biggs, Dr Mark Biggs, Sarah Biggs, Susan Biggs, Mike Edmund, Joanne Freed, Rebecca Gauntlett, Sharon Gray, Bob Herring, Mandy Howard, Caroline Howell, Becky May, Chris Miell, Gail Perry, Judith Rawlings, Jane and Nevile Reid, Arthur and Majorie Seldon, Jo Southgate, Gillian and Michael Storkey, Elaine Tanner, John and Jayne Wright, and of course our families for their continued support and patience.

In addition, our thanks go to: Eastern Energy (TXU), Australia; Lung and Asthma Information Agency, London, UK; Pollen Research Unit, Worcester, UK; and RoomService, London, UK.

Last, but not least, our grateful editorial thanks go to: Jonathan Hilton and Casey Horton for copy-editing; Selina Mumford and Julia North for project management; Helen Stallion for picture research; and Judith More, our executive editor.

Anita Reid and Dr Peter Howarth
January 2000